Systemic Sclerosis

Systemic Sclerosis

An Illustrated Guide to Manifestation and Management in Asian Skin

Edited by

Aparna Palit

Arun C. Inamadar

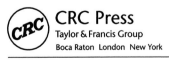

CRC Press
Taylor & Francis Group
Boca Raton London New York

CRC Press is an imprint of the
Taylor & Francis Group, an **informa** business

CRC Press
Taylor & Francis Group
6000 Broken Sound Parkway NW, Suite 300
Boca Raton, FL 33487-2742

© 2019 by Taylor & Francis Group, LLC
CRC Press is an imprint of Taylor & Francis Group, an Informa business

No claim to original U.S. Government works

Printed on acid-free paper

International Standard Book Number-13: 978-1-1384-8004-9 (Hardback)

Library of Congress Cataloging-in-Publication Data

Names: Palit, Aparna, editor. | Inamadar, Arun C., editor.
Title: Systemic sclerosis : an illustrated guide to manifestation and management in Asian skin / [edited by]
    Aparna Palit, Arun C Inamadar.
Other titles: Systemic sclerosis (Palit)
Description: New York, NY : CRC Press/Taylor & Francis Group, [2019] |
Includes bibliographical references and index.
Identifiers: LCCN 2018049601 | ISBN 9781138480049 (hardback : alk. paper) | ISBN 9781351063944 (ebook)
Subjects: | MESH: Scleroderma, Systemic | Asian Continental Ancestry Group | Atlases
Classification: LCC RC924.5.S34 | NLM WR 17 | DDC 616.5/44--dc23
LC record available at https://lccn.loc.gov/2018049601

Visit the Taylor & Francis Web site at
http://www.taylorandfrancis.com

and the CRC Press Web site at
http://www.crcpress.com

Contents

Foreword

Systemic sclerosis is a rare and complex multisystemic disease whose management most closely involves a dermatologist and rheumatologist. As cutaneous involvement is the earliest and most frequent manifestation of scleroderma, the illustrations from this book will equip the readers for an early and correct diagnosis. With recent advances in understanding of scleroderma, it is evident that early diagnosis before the end organ manifestations occur improves clinical outcomes. I can think of no better way to learn about varied cutaneous presentations than by studying the pictorial monograms.

This monogram is edited by Dr. Aparna Palit and Dr. Arun Inamadar, both leaders and highly respected authorities in this field, who have recruited a stable of experts to contribute to this valuable resource. Writing specifically about manifestations of scleroderma in Asians, the authors draw upon their extensive experience of treating scleroderma patients and providing up-to-date, practical information that will help doctors manage these patients' conditions better and improve their quality of life.

The guide begins with an easily accessible description of the basic pathogenesis. An extensive pictorial depiction of the clinical features of scleroderma and similar diseases helps readers distinguish between the many manifestations of the disease. Equally importantly, authors have incorporated the latest updates from the field. The book concludes with a discussion about complex topics such as juvenile onset scleroderma and overlap syndromes. The editors' and authors' compassion and dedication to caring for patients with scleroderma is evident throughout the book.

This is a comprehensive but easy-to-read book that I recommend every medical practitioner read and keep on hand as a reference. Touching on virtually every aspect of this disorder, *Systemic Sclerosis: An Illustrated Guide to Manifestation and Management in Asian Skin* provides a reliable source of information appropriate for all practitioners.

Pravin Patil, MRCP (UK), CCT (Rheum)
Consultant Rheumatologist
Pune, India

Preface

Systemic sclerosis is an autoimmune collagen vascular disorder characterized by fibrosis of the skin and internal organs and widespread vasculopathy. Though uncommon, it is associated with high morbidity and mortality. Improved understanding of systemic sclerosis has allowed better management of the disease. In this monogram the clinical features of systemic sclerosis from dermatologists' perspectives and the best approaches for its management have been discussed.

Systemic Sclerosis: An Illustrated Guide to Manifestation and Management in Asian Skin is an attempt to bring in all the updated information about the disease. The highlight of the book is pictorial depiction of all the relevant skin manifestations of the disease in Asian brown skin. It's easier to understand a picture than to read and process words on a page (Da Vinci's reason for favoring images over words).

This monogram has a proven hallmark features; a lucid presentation of the chapters, addition of relevant pictorial examples (more than 70), and scores of tables, flow charts, and boxes (almost 50 in total). Subject discussion is kept at a level to cater to the needs of undergraduate and postgraduate students, practicing dermatologists, and dermatologists and rheumatologists working in academic institutions.

We hope that this book provides all the necessary scientific information on systemic sclerosis for the better understanding and optimal patient care.

We sincerely thank all the contributing authors for their exceptional academic input. We thank the CRC Press publishers for all the help during the process of compiling the book and the excellent printing.

We wish to thank our readers in advance and appreciate any suggestions, comments, and corrections for the future editions of the monogram.

Aparna Palit
Arun C. Inamadar

Editors

Dr. Aparna Palit, MD (Dermatology, Venereology, and Leprology) has done her postgraduate residency at the Postgraduate Institute of Medical Education and Research (PGIMER), Chandigarh, India. Currently, she is professor and head of the Department of Dermatology and Venereology AIIMS, Bhubaneshwar, Odisha, India.

Dr. Palit has more than 100 publications to her credit. She has edited six books and written about 40 chapters in the textbooks of the speciality. She was assistant editor of the *Indian Journal of Dermatology, Venereology & Leprology* (2014–2016). She has been a reviewer of various journals: *Leprosy Review*, *British Journal of Dermatology*, *Indian Journal of Dermatology, Venereology & Leprosy*, *Indian Journal of Pediatric Dermatology*, *Indian Journal of Dermatology*, *Indian Journal of Sexually Transmitted Diseases* and *Pigment International*.

She has been awarded with the Professor L.K. Bhutani Memorial Award for Teaching and Research in 2012, and she is the recipient of the Professor R. Shivkumar & K. Rajendran Oration, IADVL-KN, 2016.

Her areas of interest include leprosy, pediatric dermatology, and collagen vascular disorders.

Arun C. Inamadar, MD, DVD, FRCP (Edinburgh) is professor and head of the Department of Dermatology, Shri BM Patil Medical College, Hospital and Research Center, BLDE University, Vijayapur, Karnataka, India.

He is a dedicated academician with more than 150 published articles; he has contributed more than 50 chapters in various textbooks and edited eight books in Dermatology. He has presented papers and delivered guest talks in several national and international scientific meets.

His path-finding work on cutaneous manifestations of "Chikungunya fever" and detailed review on the concept of "acute skin failure" is well-known in global dermatology literature. His contribution to the development of the pediatric dermatology subspecialty in India is acknowledged.

Dr. Inamadar has served as vice president of the Indian Association of Dermatology, Venereology, and Leprology (IADVL) and as the chairperson of IADVL Academy of Dermatology. He is a Fellow of the Royal College of Physicians (FRCP) from Edinburgh, UK. He has been awarded the WHO fellowship in HIV/AIDS (USA), IADVL-GlaxoSmithKline Oration (2009), and the Professor L.K. Bhutani Memorial Award for Teaching and Research (2011).

He has served as associate editor at the *Indian Dermatology Online Journal* (2011–2012) and member of the editorial board of IJDVL. Currently, he is the section editor (genotrichology) of *International Journal of Trichology*, co-editor of the *IADVL Textbook of Dermatology* (4th Edition), a member of the editorial boards of the *Indian Journal of Pediatric Dermatology* (IJPD), the *Indian Journal of Study of Sexually Transmitted Diseases*, and the *Indian Journal of Drugs in Dermatology*, and chief editor of *Clinical Dermatology Review*.

His areas of interest include clinical/medical dermatology, pediatric dermatology, and critical care in dermatology.

Contributors

Keshavmurthy A. Adya
Department of Dermatology, Venereology, and Leprosy
Shri B M Patil Medical College Hospital and Research Center
BLDE University
Vijayapur, India

Arun C. Inamadar
Department of Dermatology, Venereology, and Leprosy
Shri B M Patil Medical College, Hospital and Research Center
BLDE University
Vijayapur, India

Ajit B. Janagond
Department of Dermatology, Venereology, and Leprosy
Shri B M Patil Medical College Hospital and Research Center
BLDE University
Vijayapur, India

Akanksha Kaushik
Department of Dermatology, Venereology, and Leprology
Postgraduate Institute of Medical Education and Research
Chandigarh, India

M. Sendhil Kumaran
Department of Dermatology, Venereology, and Leprology
Postgraduate Institute of Medical Education and Research
Chandigarh, India

Rahul Mahajan
Department of Dermatology, Venereology, and Leprology
Postgraduate Institute of Medical Education and Research
Chandigarh, India

Aparna Palit
Department of Dermatology and Venereology
AIIMS, Bhubaneswar
Odisha, India

S. Ragunatha
Department of Dermatology, Venereology, and Leprosy
ESI Medical College and Hospital
Bangalore, India

Muhammed Razmi T.
Department of Dermatology, Venereology, and Leprology
Postgraduate Institute of Medical Education and Research
Chandigarh, India

Systemic sclerosis: An overview

APARNA PALIT AND ARUN C. INAMADAR

INTRODUCTION

Systemic sclerosis (SSc), or scleroderma, is a unique collagen vascular disorder characterized by variable degree of dermal fibrosis. The resulting skin hardening gives rise to a typical set of tell-tale changes in patient's appearance that are evident to the clinicians and other regular onlookers as well.[1] All patients with advanced scleroderma bear a look-alike face making it easy to identify the disorder from a distance. The associated impaired quality of life and morbidity are devastating for the patient, and the progressive course of the disease, in spite of all treatment modalities, are wearisome for the clinicians.

HISTORICAL PERSPECTIVES

Historically, the patients described by Hippocrates with "hard, parched and sweat-less skin" probably suffered from SSc.[1,2] Italian physician Giovambattista Fantonetti was the first to coin the term "scleroderma" (1836), though the evolution of the disease in his description does not tally well with this disorder.[1] By the end of nineteenth century, scleroderma was a clinically well-recognized disorder among the physicians with cutaneous and systemic involvement.[1] Sir William Osler[3] aptly compared the gradual withering and wasting of patients suffering from scleroderma to the appearance of the Greek mythological figure Tithonus, who was gifted immortality without everlasting youth.[1,4]

EPIDEMIOLOGY

SSc is ubiquitous affecting people of any race, though gender and geographical location-wise variations have been observed. The reason for an apparent increase in the incidence of SSc in recent epidemiological studies may be manifold; newer, more sensitive and specific diagnostic criteria, improved diagnostic techniques, and better understanding of the pathogenesis of the disease.[5,6]

In several epidemiological studies from different regions of the United States (published 1971–2008), the incidence rate of SSc was <2/million populations and the prevalence rate was >25 cases/million populations.[7] In another, a US healthcare claims database (2003–2008) study, where age and gender-adjusted patient data was estimated, incidence and prevalence of systemic sclerosis were 5.6 and 13.4–18.4 cases/100,000 populations, respectively.[7] Currently, the US has the highest prevalence rate for SSc (276 cases/million inhabitants) followed by Australia (233 cases/million inhabitants).[5]

European countries have a lower incidence rate as compared to the US; a higher prevalence of the disease has been found in southern European countries as compared to northern.[6] In a rheumatologists-assessed epidemiological study on SSc patients (2014) conducted in Brazil, the incidence rate was found to be 11.9%/million habitants and the prevalence rate was 105.6%/million inhabitants.[5] An incidence rate of 7.2% and a prevalence of 38%–53% has been reported from a Japanese study (1987).[8] Other Asian countries, like Taiwan and India, also have a lower prevalence of SSc.[9–11]

Various authors have reported a region-wise higher prevalence of the disease in a given country. Such variations were attributed to the high frequency of susceptibility to HLA- haplotypes (HLA-B51 and HLA-DR2) among the inhabitants as well as the level of exposure to silica-dust.[6,12–14]

A higher incidence, earlier onset, and greater severity of the disease has been recorded among black races.[6] Females are more common sufferers than males (7:1).[6] A higher occurrence among females (9.7:1) was recorded in the Italian population.[15,16] The reason for gender predilection is unknown; influence of estrogen, oral contraceptives, pregnancy, early menarche, or reproductive history do not appear to have a direct relation to the higher occurrence of the disease in women.[6] However, though men suffer from a more severe disease and show worse laboratory parameters, the Health Assessment Questionnaire with Disability Index (HAQ-DI) was found to be lower as compared to women.[17]

Currently, the pathogenesis of systemic sclerosis remains unclear. There are emerging evidences that SSc is a multi-factorial disorder. Genetic predisposition, immune deregulation, and influence of exogenous factors in variable combinations are involved in the evolution of the disease.[2]

Various environmental exposures may have direct bearing in the disease occurrence. Occupational exposure to silica and various organic solvents have been extensively studied. Men working in stone queries and gold mines have a higher risk of developing the disease.[18,19] Other occupations in textile industries, professional cleaning, film developing, medical laboratories, and publishing press may have similar higher risk of developing the disease in both males and females.[18,19] A higher risk of occurrence of SSc and other collagen vascular disorders among silicone breast implant users has not been evidenced.[20] Smoking does not contribute to the risk of occurrence of SSc but may increase the severity of the disease.[16]

Historical cases of probable scleroderma reported undergoing various therapeutic interventions like purging, bathing in hemlock water, and ingesting bittersweet.[1] Phlebotomies, vapor bath, and quicksilver were also tried.[1] Therapy of SSc has since undergone revolutionary changes with improved disease outcomes. At the end of last century, D-penicillamine was the major drug used as an anti-fibrotic agent.[21] Currently, a wide array of immunosuppressive agents is used for this purpose. Inhibition of the pro-fibrotic pathways by targeted therapy with monoclonal antibodies is on the way. Present therapeutic interventions in patients with SSc are more organ-specific to prevent complications; early therapeutic intervention with angiotensin-converting enzyme inhibitors has reduced the mortality pertaining to scleroderma renal crisis significantly.[21]

The survival rate in patients with SSc has increased over the years—from 54% in 1970s to 64% in 1990s.[22] This may be related to better diagnostic criteria leading to early diagnosis, identification of the risk factors, and increasing availability of the effective therapeutic agents over the years. Earlier, the leading cause of death in patients with SSc was "scleroderma renal crisis (SRC)." With better understanding of the precipitating factors for SRC and prophylactic therapeutic interventions, this complication is rarer now a day. However, interstitial lung disease and pulmonary arterial hypertension have taken the forefront, causing great morbidity and mortality to the patients suffering from SSc. The future directions in the research of SSc should be focused at prevention and better management of the pulmonary complications.

REFERENCES

1. De Silva U, Parish LC. Historical approach to scleroderma. *Clin Dermatol* 1994;12:201–205.
2. David M. A case of scleroderma mentioned by Hippocrates in his aphorisms. *Koroth* 1981;8:61–63.
3. Osler W. On diffuse scleroderma; with special reference to diagnosis, and to the use of the thyroid-gland extract. *J Cutan G-U Dis* 1898;16:49–67, 127–134.
4. Victorian poet Lord Tennyson. Available at https://en.wikipedia.org/wiki/Tithonus_(poem). Accessed on June 8, 2018.

5. Horimoto AMC, Matos ENN, da Costa MR et al. Incidence and prevalence of systemic sclerosis in Campo Grande, State of Mato Grosso do Sul, Brazil. *Rev Bras Rheumatol* 2017;57:107–114.

6. Nikpour M, Stevens WM, Herrick AL, Proudman SM. Epidemiology of systemic sclerosis. *Best Pract Res Clin Rheumatol* 2010;24:857–869.

7. Furst DE, Fernandes AW, Iorga SR, Greth W, Bancroft T. Epidemiology of systemic sclerosis in a large US managed care population. *J Rheumatol* 2012;39:784–786.

8. Tamaki T, Mori S, Takehara K. Epidemiological study of patients with systemic sclerosis in Tokyo. *Arch Dermatol Res* 1991;283:366–371.

9. Barnes J, Mayes MD. Epidemiology of systemic sclerosis: Incidence, prevalence, survival, risk factors, malignancy and environmental triggers. *Curr Opin Rheumatol* 2012;24:165–170.

10. Kuo CF, See LC, Yu KH et al. Epidemiology and mortality of systemic sclerosis: A nationwide population study in Taiwan. *Scand J Rheumatol* 2011;40:373–378.

11. Minz RW, Kumar Y, Amand S. Antinuclear antibody positive antibody disorders in North India: An appraisal. *Rheumatol Int* 2012;32:2883–2888.

12. Silman A, Howard Y, Hicklin A, Black C. Geographical clustering of scleroderma in south and west London. *Rheumatology (Oxford)* 1990;29:92–96.

13. Valesini G, Litta A, Bonavita MS et al. Geographical clustering of scleroderma in a rural area in the province of Rome. *Clin Exp Rheumatol* 1993;11:41–47.

14. Englert H, Joyner J, Bade R et al. Systemic scleroderma: A spatiotemporal clustering. *Intern Med J* 2005;35:228–233.

15. Monaco AL, Bruschi M, Corte RL, Volpinari S, Trotta F. Epidemiology of systemic sclerosis in a district of northern Italy. *Clin Exp Rheumatol* 2011;29(Suppl 65):S10–S14.

16. Barnes J, Mayes MD. Epidemiology of systemic sclerosis: Incidence, prevalence, survival, risk factors, malignancy, and environmental triggers. *Curr Opin Rheumatol* 2012;24(2):165–170.

17. Nashid M, Khanna PP, First DE. Investigators of the D-penicillamine, human recombinant relaxin and oral bovine type I collagen clinical trials. Gender and ethnicity differences in patients with diffuse systemic sclerosis: Analysis from three large randomized clinical trials. *Rheumatology (Oxford)* 2011;50:335–342.

18. McCormic ZD, Khuder SS, Aryal BK, Ames AL, Khuder SA. Occupational silica exposure as a risk factor for scleroderma: A meta-analysis. *Int Arch Occup Environ Health* 2010;83:763–769.

19. Bovenzi M, Barbone F, Pisa FE et al. A case control study of occupational exposures and systemic sclerosis. *Int Arch Occup Environ Health* 2004;77:10–16.

20. Janowsky EC, Kupper LL, Hulka BS. Meta-analyses of the relation between silicone breast implants and the risk of connective-tissue diseases. *N Eng J Med* 2000;342:781–790.

21. Boin F, Wigley FM. Clinical features and treatment of scleroderma. In: Firestein GS, Budd RC, Gabriel SE, McInnes IB, O'Dell JR, Eds. *Kelley's Textbook of Rheumatology*, Vol. 2, 9th ed. Philadelphia, PA: Elsevier Saunders, 2013, pp. 1363–1403.

22. Steen VD, Medsger TA. Changes in the causes of death in systemic sclerosis, 1972–2002. *Ann Rheum Dis* 2007;66:940–944.

2

Pathogenesis

S. RAGUNATHA

INTRODUCTION

The pathogenesis of systemic sclerosis (SSc) is extremely complex and heterogeneous. The characteristic pathological changes that occur in SSc are progressive cutaneous and visceral fibrosis, obliteration of small arteries and arterioles, and production of tissue-specific autoantibodies.[1] Extensive research on vasculature, immune response, cytokine profile and fibroblasts (FB) has enabled understanding of major components of pathogenesis of SSc. These include imbalance of immune response, vascular dysfunction, and activation of resident connective tissue cells.[2]

The pathogenesis of SSc is a result of interplay between epithelial, endothelial, immunological, and mesenchymal cells in a genetically susceptible individual orchestrated by secreted cytokines and growth factors through autocrine or paracrine effects. These mediators are secreted by more than one group of cells and act on multiple targets leading to a series of events responsible for development and persistence of vascular injury and fibrosis.[3] However, the unifying mechanism explaining the cascade of events resulting into characteristic pathological and clinical manifestations of SSc remains uncertain.[4]

SUSCEPTIBILITY FACTORS

Ethnicity and race

Several population-based studies have established the association of ethnicity with development and severity of SSc. The disease occurrence is higher in Choctaw Native Americans and Blacks. There is a younger age of onset, higher frequency of diffuse skin involvement, pulmonary disease, and overall worse prognosis in Black individuals as compared to Whites. The Hispanic and Native Americans develop a more severe disease than Whites. Anti-centromere antibodies are commonly found in Whites, and anti-ribonucleoprotein and anti-fibrillarin antibodies are common in Blacks. Anti-Scl70 antibodies are found in equal frequency in all ethnic groups.[5]

Genetic factors

Genetic factors not only influence susceptibility, but also predispose an individual to develop different clinical phenotypes of SSc. The observations made in family and ethnic groups of SSc patients strongly suggest the role of genetic factors in determining the susceptibility of an individual to develop the disease (Box 2.1).[6]

The inherited genetic factors mostly determine the production of autoantibodies but are not sufficient for the development of the disease. This fact has been supported by the observations made in identical twins, where the concordance for the presence of specific antibodies was substantially higher as compared to the non-significant concordance of the occurrence of SSc (4.2%).[1] The de novo alterations in loci near the Secreted Protein Acidic and Rich in Cystein (SPARC), fibrillin-1 (FBN-1), major histocompatibility complex (MHC), and TOPO-1 genes have shown significant association with SSc in the Choctow population. However, further studies in other populations would facilitate understanding the association between de novo DNA alterations and the occurrence of SSc.[6]

Human leukocyte antigen (HLA) association

Several HLA and non-HLA gene have shown consistent association with the occurrence of SSc and autoantibody profile in different ethnic groups (Table 2.1). The HLA association do not completely account for the occurrence of SSc. In a familial study, the first degree relatives showing the same HLA haplotype similar to that of the SSc patient did not develop the disease.[6]

Single nucleotide polymorphism (SNP)

Several linkage and association studies have demonstrated the association of single nucleotide polymorphisms in different genes and SSc (Box 2.2).[7]

Dinucleotide repeats at upstream region of COL1A2, SNP at codon 10 of transforming growth factor-beta (TGF-β) gene, and SNP at upstream region of Fibrillin-1 gene have been demonstrated in patients with SSc. These abnormalities have shown to increase the activity of the respective genes that are associated with fibrosis.[1] In animal models, none of the polymorphisms have shown to play a causative role. However, certain SNPs are more likely to direct the phenotypic presentation in susceptible individuals (Box 2.3).[6]

BOX 2.1: Evidences favoring the role of genetic factors[1,6]

- Female preponderance
- Familial cases
- HLA-association with SSc-associated autoantibodies
- Association with polymorphism
- Increased prevalence of anti-nuclear antibody (ANA) in first degree relatives
- Increased concordance for the presence of ANA in monozygotic twins discordant for SSc
- Gene expression profiling of fibroblasts shows a SSc molecular fingerprint in monozygotic twins discordant for SSc

Table 2.1 Common associations between HLA-class II and non-HLA genes and SSc in different ethnic groups

Sl. no.	Genes	Ethnic group	Remarks
1	HLA-DRB1 * 11	Choctaw Native Americans, Whites, Blacks, Hispanics, Japanese	Associated with Anti-topoisomerase 1 antibody
2	HLA-DRB1 * 0301	Whites in UK	
3	HLA-DQB1 * 0301	Whites, Blacks and Hispanics from Texas, and Choctaw Native Americans	
4	HLA-DRB1 * 1602	Choctaw Native Americans	Associated with Anti-topoisomerase 1 antibody
5	HLA-DRB1 * 1502	Japanese	Associated with Anti-topoisomerase 1 antibody
6	HLA-DRB1 * 0803	Japanese	
7	FBN1	Choctaw Native Americans, Japanese	Among 5 SNPs identified, 2 are specific for SSc
8	SPARC	Choctaw Native Americans, Whites and Hispanics	Homozygotes for C-allele at SNP +998 increased in Hispanics and Choctaw Native Americans

Source: Reveille, J.D., Curr. Rheumatol. Rep., 5, 160–167, 2003.
Abbreviations: FBN: Fibrillin-1, HLA: Human leukocyte antigen, SNP: Single nucleotide polymorphism, SPARC: Secreted Protein Acidic and Rich in Cystein.

BOX 2.2: Single nucleotide polymorphism in different genes associated with SSc[7]

1. Connective Tissue Growth Factor (CTGF)
2. Signal Transducer and Activator of Transcription 1 (STAT4)
3. Interferon Regulatory Factor 5 (IRF5)
4. B-Cell Scaffold Protein with Ankyrin Repeats 1 (BANK1)
5. Family with Sequence Similarity 167 Member A (FAM167A)
6. T-box transcription factor 21 (TBX21)
7. Tumor Necrosis Factor Super Family Member 4 (TNFSF4)
8. Hepatocyte Growth Factor (HGF)
9. Chromosome 8p23.1-B Lymphoid Tyrosine Kinase (C8orf13-BLK)
10. Potassium Voltage-Gated Channel Subfamily A Member 5 (KCNA5)
11. Protein Tyrosine Phosphatase Non-receptor type 22 (PTPN22)
12. Nucleotide-binding domain and Leucin-rich Repeat (NLR) family Pyrin domain 1 (NLRP1)
13. Hypoxia Inducible Factor 1 A (HIF1A)
14. Sex-determining Region Y (SRY)-Box5 (SOX5)
15. Cluster of Differentiation (CD) 226, CD 247
16. Interleukin-2 Receptor Alpha Chain (IL2RA)
17. Interleukin-12 Receptor Subunit Beta2 (IL12RB2)

BOX 2.3: SNPs involved in phenotypic presentation in susceptible individuals[6]

1. Collagen type 1
2. Fibronectin
3. Interleukin-1 α
4. Interleukin-4R α
5. Interleukin-8
6. CXC receptor-2
7. Tumor necrosis factor-α and β
8. SPARC
9. Fibrillin-1
10. TGF-β
11. Glutathione-S transferase
12. Cytochrome P450
13. Angiotensin-converting enzyme (ACE)
14. Nitric Oxide synthetase
15. Tissue inhibitor of metalloprotease (TIMP)-1
16. Stromelysin/MMp-3
17. Cytotoxic T cell-associated antigen (CTLA)-4
18. Interleukin-10

Several external and internal factors (though remain inconclusive) trigger the epigenetic modifications in patients with SSc (Box 2.4). The methylation of DNA and histone is mediated by methyl donors and co-factors, which are provided by nutritional sources. The epigenetic links between pre- and early post-natal nutritional adaptations and susceptibility to chronic diseases and between nutrition and autoimmunity indicate the role of diet and nutrition in triggering epigenetic mechanisms.

Hypoxia is another important trigger resulting in the global reduction in transcriptional activity. Hypoxia induces upregulation of HDAC and consequently leads to decreased acetylation of H3K9, which is located near the promoter region of hypoxia-activated genes such as vascular endothelial growth factor (VEGF). The oxidative stress and reactive oxygen species (ROS) are implicated directly or indirectly in the pathogenesis of SSc. FBs are the endogenous source of ROS in patients with SSc independent of inflammation. The oxidative stress controls DNA methylation and involved in epigenetic regulation of gene expression.

Hence, epigenetic modifications along with genetic susceptibility and environmental factors play a critical role in delineating the pathogenesis of SSc.[7]

PATHOGENIC MECHANISM

Epigenetic mechanisms

The role of epigenetic mechanisms is being explored to understand the pathogenesis of SSc. Epigenetics control the pattern of gene expression and cell differentiation. It is a heritable change in gene expression that does not involve alterations in DNA sequence. The epigenetic mechanisms include DNA methylation and histone modifications, which modulate chromatin structure resulting in gene transcription or repression (Table 2.2). Micro RNAs (miRNA) are also considered as epigenetic mechanism as they contribute to gene expression through post-translational modifications. There is evidence to suggest that these epigenetic mechanisms involving various genes in FBs, microvascular endothelial cells (MVEC), B cells, and T cells are playing an important role in the pathogenesis of SSc.[7]

Microchimerism

The demonstration of the similarity between graft versus host disease (GVHD) and SSc with respect to clinical, histopathological, and serological features has led to the hypothesis of microchimerism. According to this hypothesis, the maternal and fetal cells cross the placenta and persist in the circulation and tissues of child and mother, respectively. These engrafted foreign cells get activated by a second event later in life and elicit graft versus host reaction presenting as SSc. The fetal DNA and cells have been demonstrated in women with SSc who gave birth to a male fetus decades before. Similarly, maternal cells have been demonstrated in the circulation of offspring explaining the occurrence of SSc in nulliparous women. The sequence of the male chromosome in women with SSc has been similar to that of controls. However, the quantity of male DNA in the skin of patients with SSc and controls shows significant difference.[1]

Table 2.2 Epigenetic mechanisms, defects and consequences

Sl. No.	Mechanism	Gene	Cell type	Normal function	Defect	Consequence
1	DNA hypermethylation	FLI1	FB	Negative regulator of collagen production in FBs	Fli-1 transcription factor expression is reduced	Increased collagen gene expression by FBs
		BMPRII	MVEC	Favors MVEC survival and apoptosis resistance	Decreased expression of BMPRII	Enhanced response of MVECs to apoptotic signals like oxidation injury
		NOS3	MVEC	NO has vasodilatation, antithrombotic, antiplatelet, and anti-oxidation properties	Reduced expression of NOS3	Impaired wound healing, angiogenesis, and neovascularization in animal model
2	DNA hypomethylation	CD70	CD4 T cell	Co-stimulatory molecule present on activated B and T cells	Increased expression of CD70	Abnormal immune response leading to autoimmune disorders like SLE
		CD11a	CD4 T cell	Adhesive interactions between T cells, dendritic cells, and B cells	Increased expression of CD11a	Abnormal immune response leading to autoimmune disorders like SLE
		CD40L	CD4+ T cell, FB	B cell activation, expression of adhesion molecules on endothelium, and fibrosis	Increased expression in CD4+ T cells and FB	B cell activation, expression of adhesion molecules on endothelium, and fibrosis are increased
3	H3 and H4 deacetylation	FL1	FB	Negative regulator of collagen production in FBs	Fli-1 transcription factor expression is reduced	Increased collagen gene expression by FBs
4	H4 hyperacetylation and H3 hypomethylation	Global	B cells	Associated with transcriptional activity	Downregulation of HDAC2 and HDAC7	Changes in chromatin resulting in increased expression of autoimmune-related genes and antibody production

Source: Altorok, N. et al., *Rheumatology*, 54, 1759–1770, 2015.
Abbreviations: BMPR: Bone Morphogenic Protein Receptor; FB: Fibroblasts, HDAC: Histone deacetylase, MVEC: Microvascular endothelial cells, NO: Nitric oxide, NOS: Nitric oxide synthase.

BOX 2.4: The factors that trigger epigenetic modifications[7]

External factors

1. Diet and nutrition
2. Chemicals
3. Exposure to silica
4. Toxins
5. Drugs

Internal factors

1. Ageing
2. Sex hormones
3. Hypoxia
4. Oxidative injury

The triggers

The triggering factors that set off the process of characteristic pathological changes in SSc remain uncertain, in spite extensive research. As in other diseases, genetic and environmental factors play a crucial role in the pathogenesis of SSc; the latter being more influential in the development of the disease. Many infectious, chemical, and physical agents have been implicated as triggering factors (Box 2.5).[1]

BOX 2.5: Inciting factors in the pathogenesis of SSc[1]

1. Infections
   a. Cytomegalo virus (CMV)
   b. Epstein-Barr virus
   c. Parvo virus B19
   d. Herpes viruses
   e. Retrovirus
2. Exposure to environmental factors
   a. Silica
   b. Organic solvents
   c. Metallic dust
   d. Pesticides
   e. Industrial fumes
   f. Hair dye
   g. Vinyl chloride
3. Genetic factors
   a. Single nucleotide polymorphism
   b. Epigenetic mechanisms

The molecular mimicry has been proposed to explain the role of infectious agents. The epitope on self-antigen may structurally mimic viral or bacterial proteins, and the antibodies produced against these proteins act against self-antigens leading to autoimmunity. There are several evidences to suggest a hypothesis that SSc is initiated by viral infections (Box 2.6). The vinyl chloride exposure clinically presents as skin thickening, Raynaud's phenomenon, and digital ulceration similar to SSc.[1]

In addition, anti-endothelial cell antibodies, anti-fibrillin antibodies, and antibodies against matrix metalloproteinases (anti-MMP)-1 and 3 induce apoptosis of related cells representing initial trigger in the pathogenesis of SSc (Table 2.3).[3]

The initial event

In SSc, the most fundamental and earliest pathological changes occur in microvascular endothelial cells (MVEC) and it is considered as primary event in the pathogenesis of SSc (Flow Chart 1).[8] It is perpetuated by several triggering factors (Box 2.7).

There are several evidences to suggest that microvascular injury is the earliest event in the pathogenesis of SSc preceding tissue fibrosis.

BOX 2.6: Evidences in favour of viral infections as triggering factors[1]

- The presence of high levels of IgA anti-human CMV antibodies in patients with SSc, positive for Scl-70 autoantibodies
- Capacity of IgA anti-human CMV antibodies to induce apoptosis in endothelial cells
- Sequence homologies between retroviral proteins and topoisomerase-1
- Induction of expression of retroviral proteins in normal human FBs result in SSc-like phenotype
- The presence of antibodies to retroviral proteins in patients with SSc

Table 2.3 Clinico-pathological correlation of autoantibodies in SSc

Sl. no.	Type of autoantibodies	Clinico-pathological correlation
1	ANA	Positive in almost all SSc patients
2	Anti-Scl 70	Indicates dSSc and high risk of interstitial lung disease (ILD). Higher concentrations are associated with severity of skin involvement and global disease activity.
3	Anti-centromere antibodies	Associated with lSSc. Indicates gastrointestinal involvement and digital ulceration, but less frequent lungs involvement
4	Anti-PM/ScL	Associated with inflammatory myopathy
5	Anti-RNA Polymerase III	Associated with renal crisis, progressive skin fibrosis and risk of malignancy, especially breast cancer
6	Anti-endothelial cell antibodies	Associated with vascular involvement, ischemic digital ulcers and alveolar-capillary impairment. Increased synthesis and release of thrombomodulin and factor VIII, and induction of endothelial cell apoptosis resulting in microvascular pathology.
7	Anti-ICAM-1 antibodies	Increased ROS and VCAM-1 leading to proinflammatory activation of endothelial cells
8	Anti-angiotensin II receptor type 1	Vascular injury and fibrosis
9	Anti-endothelin receptor type A	Vascular injury and fibrosis
10	Anti-PDGF receptor	Increased ROS

Source: Raja, J., and Denton, C.P., *Semin. Immunopathol.*, 37, 543–557, 2015.
Abbreviations: ANA: Anti nuclear antibodies, dSSc: Diffuse cutaneous systemic sclerosis, ICAM: Intercellular adhesion molecule, ILD: Interstitial lung disease, lSSc: Limited cutaneous systemic sclerosis, PDGF: Platelet derived growth factor, ROS: Reactive oxygen species, SSc: Systemic sclerosis, VCAM: Vascular cell adhesion molecule.

BOX 2.7: Triggering factors for endothelial cell injury[2,8]

1. Vasculotropic viruses
2. Inflammatory cytokines, Transforming growth factor-beta (TGF-β), Platelet derived growth factor (PDGF), Connective tissue growth factor (CTGF), and adhesion molecules
3. Granzymes
4. Reactive oxygen species
5. Endothelial cell specific antibodies

The morphological changes in vessels prior to the onset of SSc indicate that the disease is initiated in vasculature.[9] In an animal model, it has been demonstrated that the apoptosis of endothelial cells occur prior to the infiltration of inflammatory cells or deposition of extracellular matrix (ECM) proteins. Similar findings have been demonstrated from skin biopsy specimens of patients with SSc. The increased titers of anti EC-antibodies in these patients indicate the role of autoantibodies.[10] An endothelial injury may also result from antibody (IgG)–dependent cell mediated-cytotoxicity and proteolytic activities present in serum.[1]

Abnormal repair processes

Various normal repair processes and cellular responses to tissue injury are dysregulated in patients with SSc. The genetic susceptibility, epigenetic phenomenon, and environmental factors in combination result in dysfunction of immune response, endothelial repair, and FBs.[4]

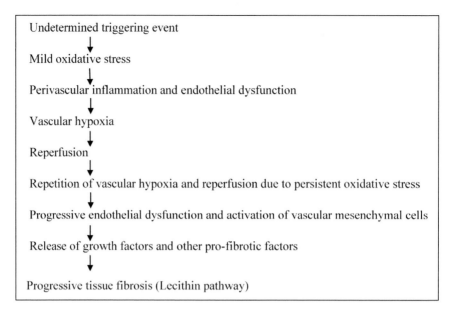

Undetermined triggering event
↓
Mild oxidative stress
↓
Perivascular inflammation and endothelial dysfunction
↓
Vascular hypoxia
↓
Reperfusion
↓
Repetition of vascular hypoxia and reperfusion due to persistent oxidative stress
↓
Progressive endothelial dysfunction and activation of vascular mesenchymal cells
↓
Release of growth factors and other pro-fibrotic factors
↓
Progressive tissue fibrosis (Lecithin pathway)

Abnormal fibrosis

In healthy individuals, fibroblasts mediate a self-limiting process of fibrosis as a part of normal tissue repair. However, in SSc, the FBs are dysregulated with inappropriate and persistent activation leading to exaggerated fibrosis. Various cytokines, chemokines, and growth factors like TGF-β and CTGF induce overexpression of genes encoding constituents of ECM like collagen (I, II, and IV), fibrillins, proteoglycans, elastin, and adhesion molecules. The oxidative stress and hypoxia can also sustain the process of fibrosis through altered inflammatory reaction.[3]

In SSc, the persistent activation of genes encoding various collagen results in uncontrolled fibrosis. However, in normal wound healing these genes are regulated resulting in controlled repair process. The transcription rate of respective genes regulates the quantity of extra cellular matrix (ECM) produced. The transcription rate, in turn, is regulated by the recognition and binding of transcription factors specifically to the nucleotide sequence at the promoter region of the concerned genes. In SSc, Spl and CCAAT-binding factor (CBF) act as important transcription factors regulating the expression of collagen genes.[1] Several transcription and inhibitory factors modulate collagen gene expression in FBs (Box 2.8). The dysfunction of these factors result in increased collagen production in SSc.[7]

Abnormal vascular repair

In SSc, the vascular remodeling is dysregulated with the upregulation of vasoconstrictor, thrombogenic, mitotic, and proinflammatory factors, and the downregulation of vasodilatory, anti-thrombogenic, and anti-mitogenic factors.[9] It leads to an imbalance in vascular tone due to the relative deficiency of vasodilators and increased levels of potent vasoconstrictor endothelin-1; this results in vascular hypoxia, subsequent endothelial injury, and ECM production maintaining the vicious cycle of endothelial injury and fibrosis.[1] The resulting vasculopathy is characterized by fibrotic intimal thickening involving all the layers of vessel wall.

In general, the vasculopathy of SSc is characterized by vasoconstriction, adventitial and intimal proliferation, inflammation, and thrombosis. The fibrosis generally begins in the media of medium-sized arteries and then extends into intima and adventitia.[9] The characteristic fibrotic intimal hyperplasia causes narrowing of the vascular lumen and loss of vascular elasticity with subsequent ischemic changes like hypoxia, necrosis, and loss of tissue.[2] Impaired secretion of vasodilators, e.g., prostacyclin, nitric oxide, calcitonin-gene related peptide (CGRP), and secretion of potent vasoconstrictor ET-1 by endothelial cells further contribute to the vascular hypoxia.[3] The acute and chronic endothelial injury result in downstream events like recruitment and adherence of platelets and activation of fibrinolytic pathways.[2]

The vasculopathy in patients with SSc shows some organ-specific features. The plexiform lesions comprising of endothelial cells and myofibroblasts are common in pulmonary arterial hypertension. In scleroderma renal crisis, the renal arteries are characterized by endothelial proliferation and deposition of scar. Progressive occlusion of blood vessels due to abnormal vascular remodeling is typically seen in digital ulcerations.[9] The vasculopathy of SSc is caused by impaired vascular remodeling resulting from dysregulated angiogenesis and defective vasculogenesis.[11]

Abnormal angiogenesis

In patients with SSc, angiogenesis is insufficient. The defective angiogenesis is inadequate to overcome the tissue hypoxia associated with endothelial injury. The altered morphology of capillaries such as reduced density, microhemorrhages, and giant and bushy capillaries indicate unsuccessful attempt of angiogenesis.[10] The repeated endothelial injury leads to tissue ischemia secondary to vascular tone dysfunction and loss of capillary bed. Vascular endothelial growth factor (VEGF), one of the potent angiogenic factors is overexpressed throughout the epidermis and dermis including FBs and perivascular cells. However, the uncontrolled and chronic overexpression of VEGF in SSc is responsible for ineffective angiogenesis.

The upregulation of angiostatic factors like angiostatin and endostatin is greater than that of

angiogenic factors.[9] Epidermal growth factor-like domain 7 (EGFL7) regulates angiogenesis by promoting endothelial cell proliferation, migration, sprouting, and invasion. It plays an important role in the normal process of microvascular repair following vascular or ischemic injury. Significantly higher serum levels of EGFL7 have been reported in patients with SSc, correlating with the severity of nailfold capillary abnormalities and digital ulcers. The downregulation of EGFL7 expression on endothelial cells and mesodermal derived endothelial progenitor cells (EPC) has been demonstrated in SSc. Hence, loss of endothelial EGFL7 expression in patients with SSc plays an important role in peripheral microvascular disease and defective angiogenesis.[12]

Abnormal vasculogenesis

Vasculogenesis, the process of forming new vessels by circulating bone-marrow derived EPCs, is also defective. The reduced number of circulating EPCs has been demonstrated in SSc. The EPCs also show reduced capacity to differentiate into ECs.[10]

Abnormal immune response

The role of innate immune response has been suggested in the induction of the early phase of inflammation and stimulation of process of fibrosis.[4] The innate immune system plays an important role in the pathogenesis mediated through mast cells, NK cells, macrophages, and DCs.[3] The chronic exposure of bacterial lipopolysaccharide (LPS) causes overexpression of the Toll-like receptor (TLR)-4, co-receptors CD14, and MD2 in the lesioned skin of patients with diffuse cutaneous SSc (dcSSc). The CD14 expression can be used as a prognostic marker as it showed significant correlation with progressive and regressive skin disease. The chronic exposure of lipopolysaccharides also showed overexpression of proinflammatory chemokines, and recruitment and activation of macrophages and upregulation of TGF-β signature genes through the Toll-like receptor-4 (TLR4) activation and subsequent myeloid differentiation primary response 88 (MyD88) signaling pathway.[4]

Innate immune response recognizes the pathogen-associated molecular pattern (PAMP) via pattern recognition receptors (PRR) expressed widely on cells of immune system and FBs. TLRs, as part of circulating PRRs, play a significant role in the pathogenesis of SSc. Upon recognition of PAMPs, the TLRs stimulate the production and secretion of pro-inflammatory cytokines such as type 1 interferon (IFN), which is a regulator of innate immune system. It is produced mainly by plasmacytoid dendritic cells (DC). The dysregulation of type 1 IFN and IFN-inducible genes have been reported in patients with SSc. In the early stage of skin involvement, activated macrophages that are present around the blood vessels secrete CCL-2, TGF-β, PDGF, and INF-regulated Sialic acid-binding immunoglobulin-1 involved in the pathogenesis of SSc. The mast cells that are present around myofibroblasts in SSc also secrete inflammatory mediators like TGF-β, IL-4, IL-13, PDGF, monocytic chemotactic protein-1 (MCP-1), IFN-α, and ET-1. TGF-β secreted by mast cells, or macrophages, or the activation of TLR causes differentiation of FBs into myofibroblasts. These cells promote production of collagen leading to fibrosis. Thus, activation of innate immunity not only promotes pathogenesis, but also precedes adaptive immune response.[3]

The genome wide association studies (GWAS) identified strong association between SNPs in major histocompatibility complex (MHC) loci and SSc indicating contribution of antigen-driven adaptive immunity in the pathogenesis of SSc. However, the mechanistic effects and interaction of these genes in the pathogenesis of SSc is yet to be delineated conclusively.[13] The cell-mediated immune response through the activation of T cells also plays a role in tissue injury seen in SSc. The oligoclonal expansion of T cells observed in the lesioned skin of SSc indicates *in situ* proliferation and clonal expansion secondary to an antigen-driven response. The innate immune system stimulated by TLR is involved in activation and maturation of DCs. These cells also induce a proliferation of T cells. The immune system shows a relative shift towards a Th2 response with secretion of profibrotic cytokines, such as IL-4, IL-5, IL-6, IL-13, and MCP-1. These cytokines are also responsible for microvascular fibroproliferation and autoantibody production.[3]

Abnormal apoptosis

The differentiation of fibroblasts into myofibroblasts or activated fibroblasts is very crucial in the pathogenesis of SSc, as these cells produce ECM proteins at a higher rate. The presence of alpha-Smooth Muscle Actin (SMA) indicates a myofibroblast population. TGF-β mediates the selection of the higher number of alpha SMA positive and apoptosis resistant fibroblasts. TGF-β acts as chemoattractant to fibroblasts and protects myofibroblasts from undergoing apoptosis. TGF-β inhibits the upregulation of inducible NO synthase, a mediator of apoptosis, in IL-1 stimulated fibroblasts. The apoptosis of fibroblasts through Fas (CD95/Apo-1) signaling is also inhibited by TGF-β. Insulin-like growth factor (IGF)-1 is known to reduce non-Fas mediated apoptosis through starvation in glomerular mesangial cells, which are similar to dermal fibroblasts.

Apoptosis of myofibroblasts is very important for recovery from the inflammatory state. Cell–cell interaction is crucial in the process of apoptosis. The cell–cell interaction of fibroblasts with myofibroblasts lead to decreased activity of the latter through apoptosis mediated by IL-1 involving NO. The apoptosis is also mediated by macrophages through NO synthesis.

The lack of adhesion to substrate causes apoptosis of cells. This process is called anoikis. The fibronectin, beta-1 integrin, and other matrix proteins provide the cell–matrix adhesion required for survival of epithelial, endothelial, and mesangial cells. Hence, cell–cell and cell–matrix interaction of fibroblasts is important in the pathogenesis of SSc mediated through protection of myofibroblasts from undergoing apoptosis. In the presence of persisting inflammatory stimuli, the fibroblasts remain activated for longer period or myofibroblasts continue to produce ECM without any inhibition.[14]

Autophagy

Autophagy is a cellular homeostatic process that regulates synthesis, degradation, and recycling of cellular components. The targeted components are isolated within the autophagosomes and then fuse with lysosomes resulting in degradation or recycling. The autophagosomes are formed in response to hypoxia and starvation. The involvement of the gastrointestinal tract (GIT) in SSc results in malabsorption and malnutrition. Autophagy of mast cells has been demonstrated in patients with SSc. These patients also had GIT involvement. Autophagy plays an important role in mast cell degranulation. These mast cells that are located near blood vessels and interstitium serve as an interface between innate and adaptive immunity. The release of mediators from mast cells drives the process of fibrosis. Autophagy in non-hemopoetic cells leads to fibrosis; hence, it has been proposed to play an important role in vasculopathy and fibrosis associated with SSc.[15]

Abnormal cellular functions

Fibroblasts: Compared to normal FBs, the dermal FBs in SSc show persistent activation; produce more collagen, cytokines and chemokines; display characteristics of myofibroblasts; and exhibit increased responsiveness to cytokines and chemokines.[7] The fibroblasts maintain the structural integrity of connective tissue. The FBs in SSc are derived from mesenchymal precursor cells originating from bone marrow and tissue-specific resident cells present in surrounding tissue. These FBs are activated by mediators, such as TGF-β, CTGF, PDGF, and ET-1, and direct cell-to-cell contact. The attachment of FBs to ECM creates mechanical tension resulting in persistent activated state. In SSc, the activated FBs overproduce collagen and induce collagen-modifying enzymes.[9]

Endothelial cells: The peripheral blood of patients with SSc shows increased levels of ET-1, sICAM-1, sVCAM-1, thrombomodulin, and von Willebrand factor (vWF) indicating activation and apoptosis of endothelial cells.[10] In SSc, increased vWF levels have been reported during the initial stage of impaired control of vascular tone.[2] The initial event in the process of vasculopathy is endothelial cell activation. The exact reason for endothelial cell activation is not known, but anti-endothelial antibodies, cytomegalovirus (CMV) infection, and reactive oxygen species (ROS) have been implicated.

The persistent endothelial activation results in endothelial damage leading to apoptosis. The inability to replace apoptotic cells leads to characteristic capillary breakdown.[9] The endothelial activation leads to damage and apoptosis. These changes are detected during the early inflammatory stage, both in lSSc and dSSc. The activation of vascular endothelial cells with the release of the vasoactive mediators result in increased microvascular permeability corresponding to the early edematous phase in cutaneous manifestation of SSc. The activated endothelial cells show upregulation of vascular cell adhesion molecule-1(VCAM-1), ELAM-1, ET-1, intercellular adhesion molecule-1 (ICAM-1), and thrombomodulin. The latter three molecules are also upregulated during the apoptosis of endothelial cells. In SSc, the replacement of apoptotic endothelial cells is impaired and results in capillary breakdown. The endothelial injury not only causes vasculopathy, but also exposes sub-endothelial layers to the immune system.[2] The endothelial injury can also occur due to antibody-dependent cell-mediated cytotoxicity mediated by IgG antibodies and proteolytic activities present in serum.[1]

Several soluble markers of endothelial cell activation or damage are increased in the circulation of patients with SSc (Box 2.9).[16]

The MPs are subcellular particles. The membrane and membrane proteins of MPs reflect their cells of origin. The MPs derived from platelets, endothelial cells, and leukocytes are represented as PMPs, EMPs, and LMPs, respectively. The assay of the MPs indicates the state of their parent cells and serves as markers of inflammation and tissue damage. The micro-particles are produced and secreted following diverse biological processes (Box 2.10).[16]

In patients with dSSc, the number of cell-derived annexin-V non-binding EMPs that indicate cellular activation are increased. These are associated with markers of vascular activation, soluble E-selectins, and soluble P-selectins. However, total concentration of circulating MPs has been low in SSc. This contrasting feature may be due to increased clearance of MPs or adherence of MPs to inflamed endothelial cells.[16]

BOX 2.9: Soluble markers of endothelial activation[16]

1. ET-1
2. Intercellular Adhesion Molecule-1
3. Vascular Cell Adhesion Molecule-1
4. Thrombomodulin
5. von Willebrand Factor protein
6. P-Selectin and E-Selectin
7. Subcellular microparticles (MP)

BOX 2.10: Biological processes causing secretion of microparticles[16]

1. Cellular activation following pro-inflammatory, pro-thrombotic or pre-apoptotic stimulation
2. Exposure to high shearing stress as in severe stenosis of arteries
3. Normal cellular differentiation
4. Senescence
5. Apoptotic cell breakdown

The macrovascular endothelial dysfunction can also occur in patients with SSc. Low flow-mediated vasodilation (FMD) in brachial and coronary artery suggestive of endothelial dysfunction has been demonstrated in SSc. The patients with SSc are also at risk of atherosclerosis demonstrated by an increased intimal-medial thickness of common carotid artery in these patients, and the risk increases with age. The normal nitroglycerine mediated vasodilatation (NMD) in SSc indicates the beneficial role of early administration of vasodilatation therapy in decreasing the risk of cardiovascular disease.[17]

B-LYMPHOCYTES

B cells regulate the immune response through diverse functions, such as antigen presentation, cytokine production, lymphoid organization, differentiation of T-cells, and modulation of functions of dendritic cells. The development and progression of B cells from progenitor cells to plasma cells is tightly regulated by both positive and negative signals.[18] The altered function of B cells has been demonstrated in SSc. The abnormal B cells are responsible for polyclonal B cell activation, systemic autoimmunity, and secretion of pro-fibrotic cytokines (Flow Chart 2).[3] In SSc, the response of B cells is intrinsically abnormal. The genes related to B cells are upregulated correlating with increased infiltration of B cells in skin and lungs.

The polymorphisms involving CD19 and CD22 have been reported to increase the susceptibility to SSc. CD19, a strong positive regulator of B cells, is over-expressed in SSc.[18] In animal experiments, it has been demonstrated that the CD19 overexpression results in spontaneous antibody production.[19] It causes a breakdown of peripheral tolerance of B cells leading to autoimmunity. In the peripheral blood of patients with SSc, naïve B cells are greater in number and there is a depletion of memory B cells/early plasma cells due to apoptosis. However, overexpression of CD19 on memory B cells enhances their ability to produce immunoglobulin. Chronic activation of remaining memory B cells by CD19 leads to production of autoantibodies.[18] The autoantibodies in SSc are involved in fibrosis through activation of fibroblasts or inhibition of matrix metalloproteinases (MMP). These also target PDGF-receptor, fibrillin, MMP-1, MMP-6, endothelin Type A receptor, and angiotensin receptor. The latter two act as agonists causing vasoconstriction and fibroblast activation.[19]

On the other hand, the expression of the negative regulator CD22, which inhibits B cell receptor (BCR) signaling, is reduced on B cells. The autoantibodies against CD22 have been reported in many patients with SSc. These autoantibodies are functional and inhibit CD22 inhibitory signals.[19]

Serum-light chain immunoglobulin (sFLC) levels are markers of polyclonal B cell activation. These levels are associated with the presence and severity of skin and lung fibrosis. Increased levels of B-cell activating factor (BAFF) in the sera and skin of patients with SSc indicate B cell activation and a degree of skin involvement. Along with β-microglobulin, BAFF correlates with the severity and activity of SSc.[3] The increased expression of BAFF on B cells boosts their ability to produce IL-6 and immunoglobulins. BAFF, a potent B cell survival factor, plays an important role in the abnormal functioning of B cells. The serum level of BAFF is increased in patients with SSc and correlates with severity of SSc.

B cells also mediate fibrosis and autoantibody production by shifting immune response towards Th2 type. Activated B cells promote development of Th2 response by the production of cytokines and expression MHC class II molecules. IL-10, produced by activated B cells, inhibits the Th1 response. It also inhibits production of IL-12 by dendritic cells, a known inducer of the Th1 response. The Th2 cytokines, IL-4, IL-5, IL-6, IL-10, and IL-13 enhance antibody production by B cells. IL-4, IL-6, and IL-13 stimulate collagen synthesis by fibroblasts. In vitro studies have demonstrated that the TGF-β gene expression can be induced by IL-4 and their interaction regulates collagen gene expression. Thus, IL-4 and IL-13 along with CTGF and MCP-1 enhance the tissue fibrosis induced by TGF-β.[18]

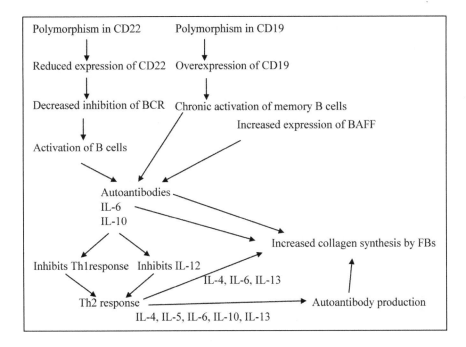

B cells also promote fibrosis by cell-to-cell contact with DCs and FBs. The regulatory B cells (Bregs) that inhibit Th1 and Th17 differentiation are deficient in SSc. Bregs also expand or maintain regulatory T cells. The number of Bregs in SSc is negatively correlated with SSc specific-autoantibodies. Bregs ameliorate autoimmune process by production of IL-10.[19]

T-LYMPHOCYTES

The presence of lymphocytic infiltration in the lesioned skin of patients with a recent onset of the disease suggests that the chronic and persistent inflammation plays an important role in the pathogenesis of the disease and it appears to be the earliest event.[1] In early skin lesions, the dermal inflammatory infiltrate is predominated by CD4+ T cells. These cells come into direct contact with MVECs and fibroblasts and result in vasculopathy and fibrosis, respectively, mediated by several profibrotic cytokines.[7] Activated CD4+ T cells form a predominant population of inflammatory cells.

In the inflammatory phase, the presence of increased serum levels of IL-2R, IL-4, TGF-β, and IL-17 indicate activation of T cells. Through these cytokines, T cells induce fibrosis. The T cells may interact with FBs via CD154/CD40 ligation to increase the production of profibrotic IL-6 and MCP-1. The T lymphocytes exhibit antigen-driven oligoclonal expansion. The candidate antigens are yet unknown; these may be foreign cells (maternal or fetal), that entered the circulation during pregnancy, CMV or topoisomerase-1. The latter exhibits several epitopes, and in patients with SSc, increased levels of CMV antigens have been reported.[20] The migration of T- lymphocytes from peripheral circulation to affected organs is mediated by expression of adhesion molecules on endothelial cells. The peripheral blood shows a reduced number of T-suppressor inducer and T-suppressor cells. It indicates imbalance between immunoregulatory T cell population. The peripheral blood of patients with SSc shows previously activated T cells indicated by spontaneous expression of high affinity IL-2 receptors (IL-2R). However, alteration in regulatory T cells and activation of T cells are results of a disease process or fundamental pathogenic event that is not yet known.[1]

Epithelial cells: In SSc, the regeneration capacity of epithelium is dysregulated. The epithelial cells secrete TGF-β and ET-1, which leads to the activation of FBs and fibrosis. The epithelial cells also undergo epithelial-mesenchymal transdifferentiation (EMT) under the influence of TGF-β and ET-1. The EMT occurs in alveolar epithelium leading to lung fibrosis.[9]

Pericytes: The pericytes also play an important part in pathogenesis of SSc. These cells are in intimate contact with endothelial cells and modulate the latter's functions. In SSc, hyperplastic and activated pericytes has been reported. They are differentiated into myofibroblasts and form a cellular link between microvascular damage and fibrosis.[9]

MEDIATORS OF PATHOGENESIS

Inflammation is a critical event that is involved in the early phase of pathogenesis and progressive vascular damage and fibrosis (Flow Chart 3).[21] Several profibrotic factors related to the peripheral immune system have been studied to describe the pathways that link inflammation and vasculopathy observed in SSc. These include TGF-β, CTGF, PDGF, and endothelin-1. Cytokines are protein mediators important for intercellular communications and regulation. These include ILs, chemokines, and cell signal molecules such as TNF-α and IFN. Various cytokines secreted by both immune and non-immune cells during the course of the disease are responsible for heterogeneous clinical manifestations of SSc.[3]

ENDOTHELIN-1

Inflammation is a critical event that is involved in the early phase of pathogenesis, progressive vascular damage and fibrosis. ET-1 is a potent vasoconstrictor over-expressed in both early and late disease. Increased levels of ET-1 in blood, lung, kidney, and skin have been demonstrated in patients with SSc. Its circulating levels have also been correlated with skin fibrosis and duration of disease. Through its action on vasculature, FBs, and inflammatory cells, ET-1 plays an important role in vasoconstriction, vascular and cardiac hypertrophy, inflammation, and fibrosis (Box 2.11).[9]

ET-1 promotes leukocyte adherence to endothelium, migration of vascular smooth muscles to intima and proliferation, and activation of perivascular fibroblasts leading to inflammation, hypertrophic and fibrotic remodeling of blood vessels, and increased synthesis of ECM, respectively.[2]

BOX 2.11: Functions of ET-1 in SSc[9]

1. Endothelial dysfunction
2. Arterial wall thickening
3. Proliferation of pulmonary arterial smooth muscles
4. Collagen production by fibroblasts
5. Down-regulation of MMP-1
6. Contraction of fibroblast-populated collagen lattice
7. Increased proinflammatory cytokines triggered by an inflammatory cascade

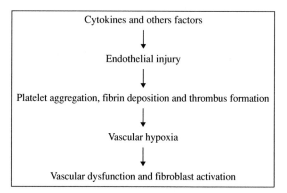

Many cells such as FBs, myofibroblasts, mast cells, macrophages/monocytes, PMNL, and dendritic cells produce ET-1 induced by hypoxia, cold exposure, low shear stress, cytokines, growth factors, and angiotensin II. TGF-β and ET-1, itself, induce production of ET-1 by FBs through the autocrine loop. ET-1 mediates its effects by binding to endothelin receptors (ETR), ET_A and ET_B present on FBs, myofibroblasts, vascular smooth muscles, and platelets. The cells of the adaptive immune system also express ETRs. B cells and PMNLs show a similar pattern of ETR expression both in SSc and healthy controls. However, higher expression of ET_A has been demonstrated on T cells and monocytes. The increased levels of ET-1, which is predominant in dSSc, suggests that ET_A preferentially mediates profibrotic effects of ET-1. Whereas increased expression of ET_B on activated CD4 T cells and CD8 T cells indicates the major role of ET_B in inflammatory effects of ET-1. Hence, the dual blockade of ETRs represents a suitable therapeutic strategy for SSc.[21]

GROWTH FACTORS

Several growth factors like TGF-β, CTGF, and PDGF play a crucial role in the fibroproliferative response seen in SSc. In patients with SSc, there is an increased expression of type I and type II TGF-β receptors on fibroblasts indicating their role in fibrosis. TGF-β promotes migration and differentiation of fibroblasts into myofibroblasts, upregulates synthesis of ECM constituents, and induces adhesions and fibrogenesis. The functions of TGF-β is mediated through various pathways, and its interaction with other cytokines has been presented in Flow Chart 4. The binding of TGF-β to its receptors triggers phosphorylation and intracellular signaling transduction resulting in the expression of genes. The downstream signaling is mediated by the SMAD family of proteins, which include activate (SMAD 1, 2, 3) and inhibitory (SMAD 7) proteins. The dysregulation of these two proteins has been demonstrated in patients with SSc. SMAD 7 is an inhibitory protein that binds to the TGF-β receptor complex and inhibits phosphorylation of stimulatory SMADs (i.e., SMAD 2 and SMAD 3); thus, inhibiting the collagen and ECM synthesis. In patients with SSc, the levels of SMAD 7 is significantly reduced resulting in unregulated and exaggerated TGF-β signaling and subsequent synthesis of collagen and ECM.[1]

CTGF demonstrates functions similar to TGF-β. Increased expression of CTGF in lesioned tissues of patients with SSc is mediated by TGF-β, hypoxia and ET-1. A variation in the promoter region of CTGF gene, which predisposes an individual to develop SSc, has been demonstrated.[3] TGF-β stimulates FBs, vascular smooth muscles, and endothelial cells to secrete CTGF. Through the autocrine loop stimulation, CTGF maintains a continuous and prolonged cycle of fibrosis by stimulating its own production.[1] The expression of another important growth factor, PDGF, is involved in fibrosis and endothelial injury and has been known to increase in the lungs, skin, and bronchoalveolar lavage fluid of SSC patients.

PDGF promotes endothelial proliferation, ECM production, and the release of profibrotic mediators like IL-6 and MCP-1. The autocrine PDGF/PDGFRα signaling loop in FBs is dependent on TGF-β and IL-1α.[3]

The process of angiogenesis is mainly regulated by VEGF. It stimulates the migration and proliferation of ECs, increases vascular permeability, and induces tube formation. In SSc, VEGF is strongly expressed in skin and its serum level is also significantly increased. The latter bears significant correlation with fingertip ulceration in patients with SSc. Even though the VEGF levels are increased in SSc, the time kinetics of its expression plays a critical role in angiogenesis. The new vessels become untenable if upregulation of VEGF is transient. A prolonged overexpression results in uncontrolled fusion of new vessels resembling disturbed capillary network.[10] Higher levels of syndecan-1 that binds to VEGF and presents them to respective receptors on endothelial cells has been demonstrated in SSc. Higher levels of syndecan-1 correlate with SSc vasculopathy, such as telangiectasia and PAH.[11]

CYTOKINES

IL-13, an immune system-derived factor, mediates fibrosis in patients with SSc. It is produced predominantly by Th2 skewed T cells. IL-13 is also produced by macrophages, mast cells, and dendritic cells. Nuocytes belonging to a group of intrinsic lymphoid cells (ILC) that are induced by IL-33 and IL-25 are also found to be a potential source of IL-13. It utilizes the IL-4 receptor complex comprising of IL-4RA and IL-3RA1 for signaling that activates STAT6 through TYK2 and JAK2. In patients with limited cutaneous SSc (lSSc) and (dSSc), the serum levels of IL-4 and IL-13 are increased. The number of cells expressing IL-13 is also increased. These cells are positive for the macrophage marker indicating that the dermal macrophages are the source of IL-13 in the lesioned skin of patients with SSc. The peripheral CD8 T cells show increased expression of IL-13 caused by the upregulation of Th2 transcription and inhibition of differentiation towards INF-γ producing Th1 cells. These cells correlate with measures of disease severity and interstitial lung disease. Increased levels of IL-13, mRNAs encoding IL-13RA1 and the IL-13 regulated gene, CCL2, correlate with inflammatory markers (CRP and ESR), the presence of SSc, and the disease severity measured by modified Rodnan Skin Score (mRSS). Hence, IL-13 plays a critical role in the inflammatory process observed in SSc. In addition, IL-13 also plays an important role in vasculopathy associated with SSc. The IL-13 levels in patients with SSc correlate positively with pulmonary arterial hypertension (PAH) and nailfold capillary abnormalities. The profibrotic property of IL-13 has been demonstrated by several animal studies using mouse models. The upstream regulation of IL-13 secretion helps in understanding the pathological events that lead to SSc. IL-13 is induced by IL-33, a broad upstream inducer that is released upon necrotic cell death. The expression of IL-33 on endothelial cells, epithelial cells, FBs and smooth muscle cells indicates that the ischemia secondary to vascular injury in SSc is responsible for IL-33 release. Inflammation and toxin-mediated tissue injury can also release IL-33. Hence, it can be proposed that the micro-environmental stressors in lesioned skin in SSc result in release of IL-33. The stimulation of IL-33 causes activation of IL-13 expression in Th2 cells, B cells and nuocytes. IL-33 also stimulates the production of IL-13 by the innate immune cells such as mast cells and basophils.[13]

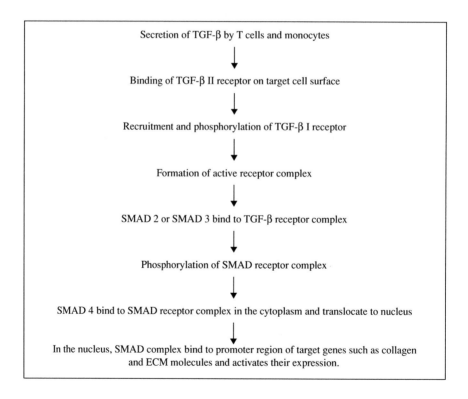

Activated T lymphocytes secrete IL-2R, IL-4, and IL-17. IL-4 and its spliced form IL-4δ2 increase the production of collagen by FBs. IL-17 has a direct effect on FBs inducing their proliferation and expression of IL-6. It also induces adhesion molecules on ECs resulting in infiltration of mononuclear cells.[20] The Th17 associated cytokines IL-17, IL-21, and IL-23 also play an important role in the pathogenesis. The increased serum levels of IL-17 correlates significantly with the lung fibrosis. IL-23 is a survival and proliferative factor for Th17 cells. Hence, exposure of Th17 cells to an antigen-presenting cell derived IL-23 is essential for induction of autoimmunity. The increased serum levels of IL-17 and IL-23 are seen in the early stages of the disease. In patients with SSc, increased levels of IL-21 has been reported. It has an angiostatic property. High IL-21 levels have been associated with development of secondary autoimmunity after alemtuzumab theray in patients with multiple sclerosis indicating its role in initiating autoimmune reactions in later stages of SSc. There have been many reports demonstrating conversion of T- regulatory cells to Th17 cells. The immunosuppressive therapy can also lead to an imbalance in Th1, Th2, Th17 and T-regulatory cell responses.[22]

CHEMOKINES

The chemokines are small molecules secreted at the focus of inflammation by sentinel cells. Chemokines are involved in early stage of pathogenesis of SSc. MCP-1 and MCP-3, belonging to the CC group of chemokines, are involved in the pathogenesis of SSc. These are expressed in mononuclear cells, fibroblasts, endothelial cells, and keratinocytes. MCP-1 and 3 promote fibrosis in the early stage of disease. The higher expression of CCL18, 19, and CXCL 13 has been reported in patients with dcSSc.[3] Increased levels of CCL18 is a result of enhanced secretion of IL-10 secreted by TLR-4 stimulated dendritic cells.[23] CCL19 expression has found to be sensitive marker of perivascular inflammation and immune cell recruitment.[3] In the inflammatory stage of the disease, MCP-1 is mainly expressed in infiltrating mononuclear cells. In late fibrotic stage, MCP-1 is expressed by fibroblasts. The expression of MCP-1 is increased in the skin of patients with SSc. The increased expression of MCP-1 in non-fibrotic skin in patients with SSc indicates its possible role in the initiation of fibrosis. The increased level of MCP-1

in blood is also demonstrated in these patients. Increased serum levels might indicate a risk of organ involvement. MCP-1 is a potent chemoattractant for mononuclear cells from the very early stages of the disease. Both MCP-1 and MCP-3 promote infiltration of inflammatory cells into the skin and subsequent stimulation of resident FBs. MCP-1 induces Th2 differentiation in Th0 cells resulting in an increased release of IL-4. MCP-3 has similar chemotactic property as that of MCP-1. Additionally, it is chemotactic for dendritic cells and granulocytes.[24]

COMPLEMENT SYSTEM

The poorly controlled complement activation in various vascular diseases has shown to promote EC damage and apoptosis, expression of vascular cell adhesion molecules, and amplification of local immune response. In patients with SSc, hypocomplementemia, and an increased complement activation has been associated with the clinical severity of the disease. The higher small vessel score of C4d is associated with an increased risk of unrecoverable renal function. Factor H (FH), a fluid-phase regulator of alternate pathway, regulates the complement activation to target only foreign agents or altered self-cells. *In vitro* studies have shown a defective capacity of FH to protect complement mediated cellular damage in patients with SSc. The impaired expression of another membrane-bound regulator, membrane regulator protein has been demonstrated in endothelium of lesioned and non-lesioned skin of patients with SSc suggesting defective endothelial protection.

SNPs in the promoter region of the MCP gene in patients with SSc may indicate more severe disease. The local activation of endothelium-bound membrane attack complex (MAC/C5b-9) has been proposed as marker of active vascular damage in SSc in the presence of normal plasma levels of complements. The sub-lethal MAC causes endothelial apoptosis leading to initiation and propagation of tissue fibrosis. The locally activated complement may affect many pathological process of SSc (Box 2.12).[25]

LEUKOTRIENES

Leukotrienes are the lipid mediators synthesized from arachidonic acid mediated by 5-lipoxygenase (5-LOX). Leukocytes are the main source of LT. LTB-4 is primarily synthesized by neutrophils,

BOX 2.12: Role of complement activation in SSc[25]

1. Vascular damage
2. Direct endothelial damage and apoptosis
3. Pro-coagulatory response
4. Lymphocyte activation
5. Recruitment of inflammatory cell
6. Fibroblast recruitment
7. Abnormal neovascularization

and cysteinyl LTs, LTC-4, LT-D-4, and LTE-4 are synthesized by eosinophils and basophils. Macrophages and monocytes secrete both LTs. These LTs regulate the process of inflammation, vascular function, and connective tissue remodeling (Table 2.4).[26]

The expression of 5-LOX is increased in patients with SSc, especially in early stages of dcSSc. These are expressed in mononuclear cells and FB-like cells throughout the skin. *In vitro* studies have demonstrated increased production of LTB-4 by FBs derived from patients with SSc. The overexpression of 5-LOX in lungs of patients with primary pulmonary hypertension indicates role of leukotriene pathway in the pathogenesis of SSc. Through activation of platelets and subsequent release of growth factors, cysteinyl leukotrienes promote fibrosis, and vascular disease in lungs.[26]

OTHER MEDIATORS

There are many mediators secreted by inflammatory cells and have been hypothesized to play role in the pathogenesis of SSc. Adipokines, chemical mediators synthesized by adipocytes, such as adiponectin, visfatin, retinol binding protein-4, apelin, and resistin, have demonstrated a potential role in the pathogenesis of SSc. Resistin, also secreted by inflammatory cells, triggers proliferative response in vascular smooth muscles resulting in angiogenesis in pulmonary vasculature. The significant increase in serum levels of resistin has been found in patients with SSc.[27]

Osteopontin, an ECM protein, demonstrates pro-inflammatory and pro-fibrotic properties. High plasma levels of osteopontin has been noted along with increased TGF-β, α-SMA levels.

Table 2.4 Functions of leukotrienes relevant to systemic sclerosis

Leukotriene B-4	• Stimulates synthesis of proinflammatory mediators like TNF-α, IL-6, IL-8 and Fibroblast growth factor
	• Recruitment of T lymphocytes through activation of macrophages and monocytes
	• Stimulates migration of fibroblasts
Cysteinyl leukotrienes	• Activation of endothelial cells
	• Increased permeability of blood vessels
	• Proliferation and migration of vascular smooth muscles
	• Synthesis of collagen
	• Differentiation of fibroblasts into myofibroblasts
	• Stimulation of synthesis of TGF-β by epithelial cells
	• Regulation of synthesis, secretion and activation of matrix metalloproteinase

Source: Chwieśko-Minarowska, S. et al., *Folia. Histochem. Cytobiol.*, 50, 180–185, 2012.

This indicates its possible role in differentiation of FBs in early stage of the disease.[28]

SUMMARY

The heterogenous nature of SSc and its prevalence in certain ethnic groups indicate the role of genetic factors in determining the susceptibility of an individual to develop the disease following exposure of appropriate triggering factors. Once initiated, the abnormal responses of endothelial cells, fibroblasts, lymphocytes, and epithelial cells secrete profibrotic cytokines and growth factors. The resulting dysregulation of vascular remodeling, angiogenesis, vasculogenesis, and immune response all culminate into characteristic pathological changes of SSc, such as fibrosis, vasculopathy, and autoimmunity. These changes correspond clinically to scleroderma, digital ischemia with nail bed capillary changes, and the presence of autoantibodies, respectively.

REFERENCES

1. Jimenez SA, Derk CT. Following the molecular pathways toward an understanding of the pathogenesis of systemic sclerosis. *Ann Intern Med* 2004;140:37–50.
2. Geyer M, Müller-Ladner U. The pathogenesis of systemic sclerosis revisited. *Clinic Rev Allerg Immunol* 2011;40:92–103.
3. Raja J, Denton CP. Cytokines in the immunopathology of systemic sclerosis. *Semin Immunopathol* 2015;37:543–557.
4. Stifano G, Affandi AJ, Mathes AL, Rice LM, Nakerakanti S, Nazari B. Chronic Toll-like receptor 4 stimulation in skin induces inflammation, macrophage activation, transforming growth factor-β signature gene expression, and fibrosis. *Arthritis Res Ther* 2014;16:R136.
5. Reveille JD. Ethnicity and race and systemic sclerosis: How it affects susceptibility, severity, antibody, genetics, and clinical manifestations. *Curr Rheumatol Rep* 2003;5:160–167.
6. Feghali-Bostwick CA. Genetics and proteomics in Scleroderma. *Curr Rheumatol Rep* 2005;7:129–134.
7. Altorok N, Almeshal N, Wang Y, Kahaleh B. Epigenetics, the holy grail in the pathogenesis of systemic sclerosis. *Rheumatology* 2015;54:1759–1770.
8. Osthoff M, Ngian G-S, Dean MM et al. Potential role of the lectin pathway of complement in the pathogenesis and disease manifestations of systemic sclerosis: A case-control and cohort study. *Arth Res Ther* 2014;16:480.
9. Abraham DJ, Krieg T, Distler J, Distler O. Overview of pathogenesis of systemic sclerosis. *Rheumatol* 2009;48:iii3–iii7.
10. Distler JHW, Gay S, Distler O. Angiogenesis and vasculogenesis in systemic sclerosis. *Rheumatology* 2006;45:iii26–iii27.
11. Ching-Ying WU, Asano Y, Taniguchi T, Sato S, Hsin-Su YU. Serum level of circulating syndecan-1: A possible association with proliferative vasculopathy in systemic sclerosis. *J Dermatol* 2016;43:63–66.
12. Manetti M, Guiducci S, Romano E et al. Decreased expression of the endothelial cell-derived factor EGFL7 in systemic sclerosis: Potential contribution to impaired angiogenesis and vasculogenesis. *Arthritis Res Ther* 2013;15:R165.
13. Greenblatt MB, Aliprantis AO. The immune pathogenesis of scleroderma: Context is everything. *Curr Rheumatol Rep* 2013;15:297.
14. Kissin E, Korn JH. Apoptosis and myofibroblasts in the pathogenesis of systemic sclerosis. *Curr Rheumatol Rep* 2002;4:129–134.
15. Frech T, De Domenico I, Murtaugh MA et al. Autophagy is a key feature in the pathogenesis of systemic sclerosis. *Rheumatol Int* 2014;34:435–439.
16. Iversen LV, Østergaard O, Ullman S et al. Circulating microparticles and plasma levels of soluble E- and P-selectins in patients with systemic sclerosis. *Scand J Rheumatol* 2013;42:473–482.
17. Szűcs G, Tímár O, Szekanecz Z et al. Endothelial dysfunction precedes atherosclerosis in systemic sclerosis—Relevance for prevention of vascular complications. *Rheumatology* 2007;46:759–762.
18. Hasegawa M. B lymphocytes: Shedding new light on the pathogenesis of systemic sclerosis. *J Dermatol* 2010;37:3–10.
19. Sakkas LI, Bogdanos DP. The role of B cells in the pathogenesis of systemic sclerosis. *Isr Med Assoc J* 2016;18:516–518.
20. Sakkas LI. New developments in the pathogenesis of systemic sclerosis. *Autoimmunity* 2005;38:113–116.
21. Elisa T, Antonio P, Giuseppe P et al. Endothelin receptors expressed by immune cells are involved in modulation of inflammation and in fibrosis: Relevance to the pathogenesis of systemic sclerosis. *J Immunol Res* 2015;2015:147616.
22. Olewicz-Gawlik A, Danczak-Pazdrowska A, Kuznar-Kaminska B et al. Interleukin-17 and interleukin-23: Importance in the pathogenesis of lung impairment in patients with systemic sclerosis. *Int J Rheumat Dis* 2014;17:664–670.

23. van Lieshout AWT, Vonk MC, Bredie SJH et al. Enhanced interleukin-10 production by dendritic cells upon stimulation with Toll-like receptor 4 agonists in systemic sclerosis that is possibly implicated in CCL18 secretion. *Scand J Rheumatol* 2009;38:282–290.

24. Distler JHW, Akhmetshina A, Schett G, Distler O. Monocyte chemoattractant protein in the pathogenesis of systemic sclerosis. *Rheumatol* 2009;48:98–103.

25. Scambi C, Ugolini S, Jokiranta TS et al. The local complement activation on vascular bed of patients with systemic sclerosis: A hypothesis-generating study. *PLoS One* 2015;10(2):e0114856.

26. Chwieśko-Minarowska S, Kowal K, Bielecki M, Kowal-Bielecka O. The role of leukotrienes in the pathogenesis of systemic sclerosis. *Folia Histochem Cytobiol* 2012;50:180–185.

27. Masui Y, Asano Y, Akamata K et al. Serum resistin levels: A possible correlation with pulmonary vascular involvement in patients with systemic sclerosis. *Rheumatol Int* 2014;34:1165–1170.

28. Corallo C, Volpi N, Franci D et al. Is osteopontin involved in cutaneous fibroblast activation? Its hypothetical role in scleroderma pathogenesis. *Int J Immunol Pharmacol* 2014;12:97–102.

3

Classification and clinical features

APARNA PALIT AND ARUN C. INAMADAR

CLASSIFICATION

The clinical picture of systemic sclerosis (SSc) may be variable at presentation. Some patients may present at the initial phase of the disease evolution with minimal skin sclerosis or only Raynaud's phenomenon, whereas others present at a later stage with the unmistakable florid, clinical picture. The classification system for SSc categorizes the entity into two subsets. The basis of this categorization is the extent of fibrosis on extremities; the limited cutaneous SSc (lSSc) and diffuse cutaneous SSc (dSSc). This categorization is of immense importance in terms of systemic involvement and disease outcome; discussed in subsequent sections. The assessment of cutaneous sclerosis is done by pinching a fold of skin on the distal extremities with two fingers of the examiner's hand (Figure 3.1) and the extent upwards is assessed.

Limited cutaneous SSc

The cutaneous sclerosis is limited to the distal extremities beyond elbows and knees, and the face is involved.[1] Trunk is spared in this subtype of the disease. A subset of patients may have sclerosis of the fingers alone for a long duration. Systemic involvement is present.

Diffuse cutaneous SSc

The skin sclerosis progresses proximal to the elbows, knees, and on the trunk.[1] Facial involvement may be absent in the initial stage of the disease. Systemic

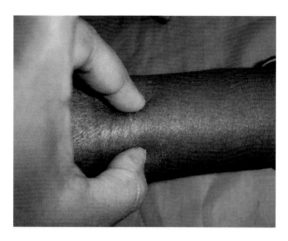

Figure 3.1 Assessment of cutaneous sclerosis.

involvement is more extensive in this subtype and carries a poor prognosis.

SSc *sine* scleroderma

There is a rare variant of SSc (1.5%) where the clinical features of cutaneous fibrosis is absent.[2,3] However, these patients have vascular (Raynaud's phenomenon) and pulmonary (pulmonary arterial hypertension) manifestations and positive anti-centromere antibodies.[2] In the absence of cutaneous sclerosis, this is designated as "SSc *sine* scleroderma."[2,3]

Scleroderma-overlap syndromes

Patients with lSSc or dSSc may have features of other collagen vascular disorders; systemic lupus erythematosus, polymyositis/dermatomyositis, Sjögren syndrome, and rheumatoid arthritis.[2] These are designated as scleroderma-overlap syndromes.

There may be a diagnostic difficulty when SSc is in evolution or the disease is minimal, as in lSSc.[3] Various classification criteria for diagnosis of SSc and sub-categorization of dSSc and lSSc have been discussed in detail in Chapter 5. These criteria are useful in diagnosis and categorization of the subsets of SSc.

CUTANEOUS MANIFESTATIONS

The predominant cutaneous involvement and the resultant clinical features can be categorized as those due to fibrosis and the others due to vasculopathy.

Cutaneous features resulting from fibrosis

Cutaneous features resulting from fibrosis volutes through two phases; the edematous phase and fibrotic phase.

EDEMATOUS PHASE

This is the initial phase, clinically characterized by non-pitting edema and mainly localized to the distal extremities and face (Figure 3.2). The patients complain of a feeling of tightness and bloating. The edema over the distal extremities may be mistaken with that of renal or cardiac origin. In rapidly progressive cases, there may be pitting edema over the involved areas (Figure 3.3). Erythema, pruritus, and

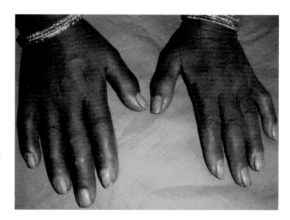

Figure 3.2 Swollen hands in the edematous phase.

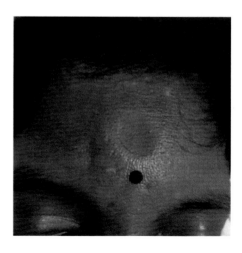

Figure 3.3 Pitting edema over the forehead and swollen eyelids during rapidly progressive edematous phase.

pain may be associated.[3] Edema localized over the wrists may give rise to pain and restriction of movements simulating carpal tunnel syndrome.[3] The edematous phase persists for few weeks, followed by a gradual transition to fibrotic phase.

FIBROTIC PHASE

During the fibrotic phase, there is a gradual sclerosis resulting in adherent, non-pinchable skin (Figure 3.4). The fibrosis is clinically appreciable over the dorsa of the hands and feet initially and, thereafter, gradually extends proximally. Cutaneous appendages are involved in the fibrotic process, clinically appreciable as dry, lustreless skin surface and sparse body hair.[3–5] This phase is gradually progressive giving rise to the classical clinical picture of PSS.

In lSSc the fibrosis is slower in onset and progression, whereas it is rapid in dSSc, reaching to maximum intensity by the initial 6–18 months.[3,5] In the advanced stage of fibrosis, the skin is shiny and taut over the face (Figure 3.5), the extremities, and over most of the bony prominences. In lSSc, it extends up to the forearms and legs (below elbows and knees), but the entire skin surface is involved gradually in dSSc. In some cases, the skin sclerosis settles down after the initial progression and may improve after the second or third year.[2]

The final effect of fibrosis on various parts of face and extremities has been discussed below.

Face and neck

Extensive fibrosis of the skin and underlying tissue results in improper contraction of the facial

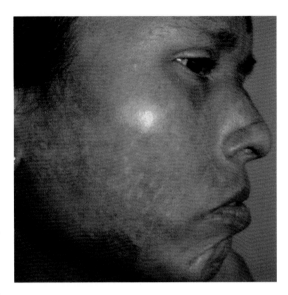

Figure 3.5 Shiny and taut skin over face during established fibrotic stage.

muscles during fine movements and loss of lines of facial expression. This gives rise to a wrinkle-less, wax-like facial skin. The ultimate effect is the "mask-facies" (Figure 3.6), very typical of patients with advanced SSc.

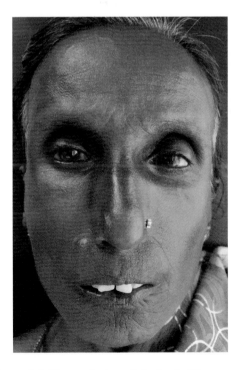

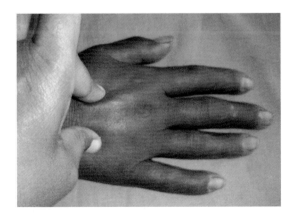

Figure 3.4 Non-pinchable skin over the dorsum of hand in fibrotic phase.

Figure 3.6 The typical mask-facies in SSc.

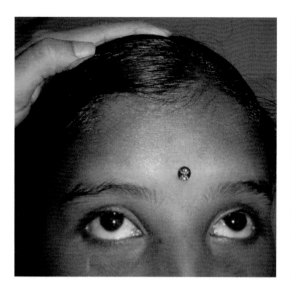

Figure 3.7 Absence of horizontal forehead lines when the patient looks up.

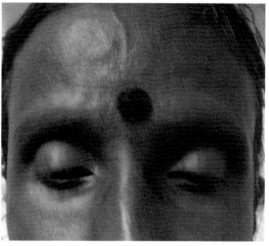

Figure 3.9 Drooping upper eyelids giving a sleepy appearance.

The horizontal lines on the forehead are not demonstrable (Figure 3.7), while the patient attempts to look upwards. The frown lines are attenuated (Figure 3.8).

In the advanced stage of sclerosis of the facial skin, the upper eyelids appear drooping giving rise to a sleepy appearance (Figure 3.9). Lower eyelids are not retractable by the clinician to look for pallor (Figure 3.10) at the palpebral conjunctiva, also known as Ingram's sign.

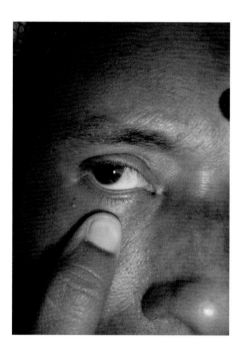

Figure 3.10 Lower eyelid is not retractable; positive Ingram's sign.

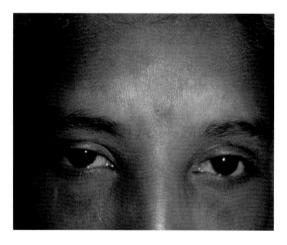

Figure 3.8 Absence of frown lines.

The bound-down skin on the cheeks, peri-nasal, and perioral areas give rise to some of the characteristic changes of scleroderma-facies.

The transverse diameter of the anterior nose, which is normally a pyramidal structure, is reduced and gives rise to a "pinched" appearance (Figure 3.11).

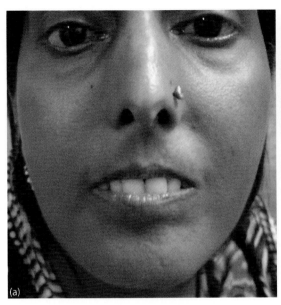

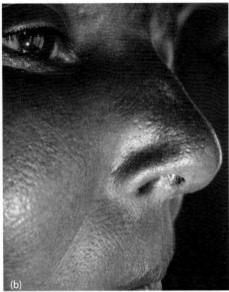

Figure 3.11 **(a, b)** Pinched appearance of the nose with narrow, oblong anterior nares.

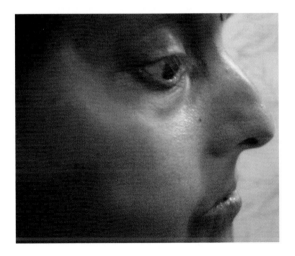

Figure 3.12 Beaked appearance of the tip of the nose.

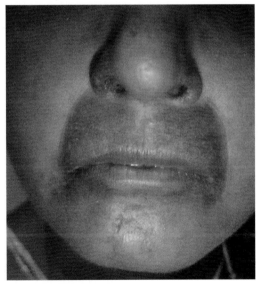

Figure 3.13 Effacement of the philtrum due to advanced fibrosis of the perioral skin.

The anterior nares become oblong and narrow, rather than the usual triangular shape. The tip of the nose is pointed forwards, which gives rise to a beaked appearance; better appreciable in side-profile (Figure 3.12). The normal concave contour of the philtrum is effaced giving rise to a flat area between

columella of the nose and vermillion border of the upper lip (Figure 3.13).

The lips are thin, and there are perioral radial furrowing giving rise to the typical purse-string appearance[5] (Figure 3.14a and b).

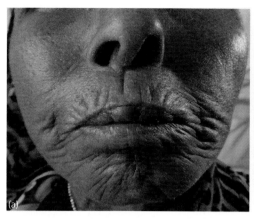
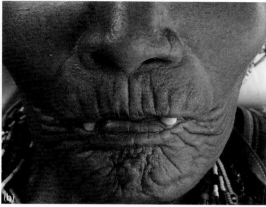

Figure 3.14 (a, b) Perioral radial furrowing with purse string appearance. Thin lips (Figure 3.14b).

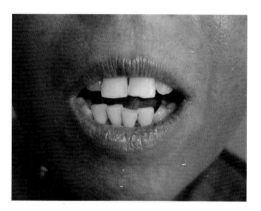

Figure 3.15 Microstomia.

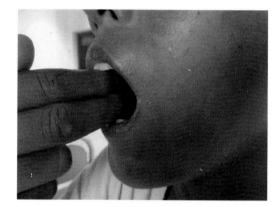

Figure 3.16 Inability to insert fingers through oral aperture in advanced microstomia.

The diameter of the oral aperture is reduced (microstomia) (Figure 3.15), so that daily activities like food intake and brushing is difficult for the patient. Clinically, it is demonstrable by insertion of the patient's fingers at a right angle through the oral aperture. Normal individuals are able to pass three fingers this way, but it is reduced in patients with SSc having advanced microstomia (Figure 3.16).

Fibrosis and tethering of the skin on mandible may lead to puckering over the chin (Figure 3.17). Dimpling may occur at the point of the chin (Figure 3.18). The normal rounded contour of the angle of the mandible is flattened (Figure 3.19), leading to overcrowding of the lower teeth (Figure 3.20).

Several changes may occur involving the structures in oral cavity. The factors contributing to the oral mucosal changes are[3,4]:

- Tightening of the facial skin
- Atrophy of the salivary glands
- Sclerosis of the oral mucosa

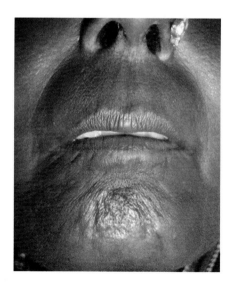

Figure 3.17 Puckering of the chin.

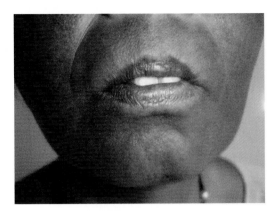

Figure 3.18 Dimpling at the point of chin.

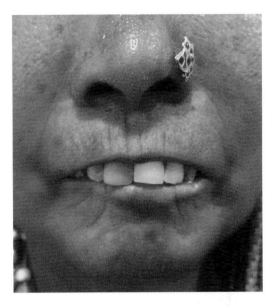

Figure 3.21 Thin lips and partly exposed upper teeth.

The oral mucosa appears dry because of decreased salivary secretion. The upper anterior teeth are partly exposed due to a thinning of the lips and gingival atrophy (Figure 3.21). Sclerosis of the frenulum (Figure 3.22) leads to restricted mobility of the tongue.[4,5]

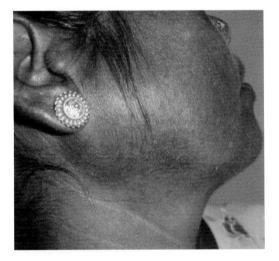

Figure 3.19 Flattening of the rounded contour of the mandible.

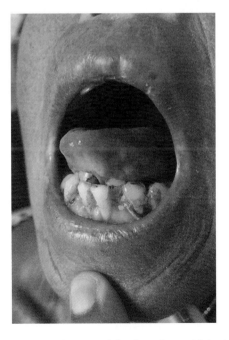

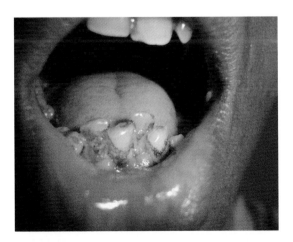

Figure 3.20 Overcrowding of the teeth in lower jaw.

Figure 3.22 Sclerosis of the frenulum with inability to protrude the tongue.

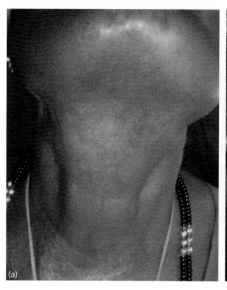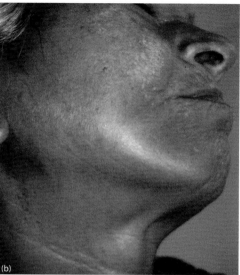

Figure 3.23 **(a, b)** Fibrotic bands on extension of the neck (Barnett's sign).

Prominent vertical fibrotic bands are visible on the front of neck in hyper-extended position, known as "scleroderma neck sign" or Barnett's sign (Figure 3.23a and b).

Hands and feet

The acral changes evolve through three overlapping phases[5]:

- Initial phase of puffy digits
- Non-pitting edema of the digits
- Rapidly progressive fibrosis resulting in sclerosis

An early symptom of the edematous phase involving the hands is an inability to remove a ring, which was loosely fitted earlier.[3] During the initial phase of fibrosis, the digits are sausage-shaped with distal tapering ends (sclerodactyly) (Figure 3.24). The extension of fibrosis to the subcutaneous tissue and fascia leads to bound down, shiny, and taut skin over the dorsa of hands and feet (Figure 3.25). The dorsal and palmar interphalangeal creases are reduced and, gradually, completely effaced in the advanced stage of fibrosis (Figure 3.26a and b).

The digits are initially, partially flexed at the interphalangeal joints (Figure 3.27). The patients may experience coarse cracking and crepitations around such joints due to involvement of the peri-articular tissues.[2,3,5] In the late fibrotic phase, there are flexion contractures of these joints (dermatogenous

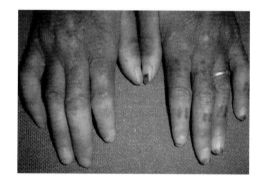

Figure 3.24 Distal tapering of the fingertips (sclerodactyly). Prominent pallor of the fingers indicates Raynaud's phenomenon.

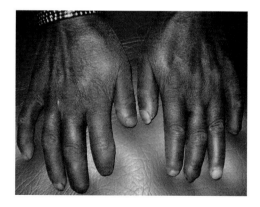

Figure 3.25 Bound down shiny skin over the dorsa of hands. Loss of distal part of the digits due to vasculopathy.

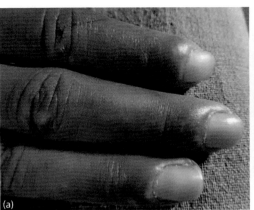
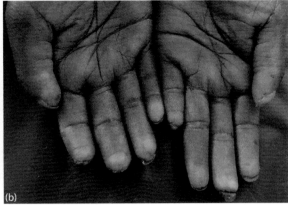

Figure 3.26 **(a, b)** Effacement of the dorsal and palmar distal interphalangeal creases.

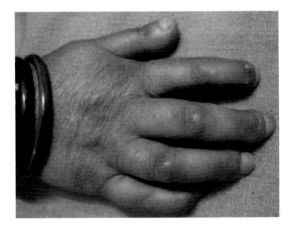

Figure 3.27 Partial flexion of the interphalangeal joints.

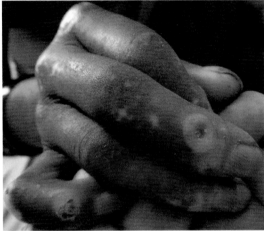

Figure 3.28 Fixed contracture of the hand with ulceration over the interphalangeal joints.

contractures).[2] The skin overlying these contracted inter-phalangeal joints may become relatively avascular and fibrotic, and traumatic ulcers may develop over these areas due to friction (Figure 3.28).[3,4]

Chest

Restricted breath excursion is a feature of cutaneous sclerosis over the trunk. Following full expiration, the patient is asked to take full inspiration; expansion of <5 cm is indicative of restricted chest movement.[6]

Pigmentary changes

Patchy or diffuse hyper-pigmentation of the fibrotic skin occurs in patients with PSS. The classical pigmentary change is the speckled hyper- and hypo-pigmentation (salt and pepper pigmentation), mostly seen over the face and neck (Figure 3.29a and b).

Telangiectasia

Telangiectasia are erythematous, macular, blanchable skin lesions of vascular origin arising from dilated post-capillary venules, without evidence of any inflammation or obstruction of vessel wall. The lesions may be isolated or coalesced. Mat-like telangiectasia are described as a flat, rectangular collection of tiny blood vessels particularly distributed over the bilateral cheeks (Figure 3.30a and b). The lesions are better appreciable in fair-skinned

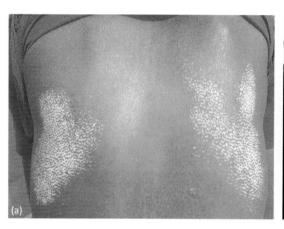
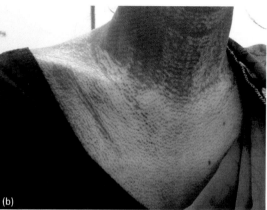

Figure 3.29 **(a, b)** Speckled "Salt and pepper" pigmentation of the trunk and neck.

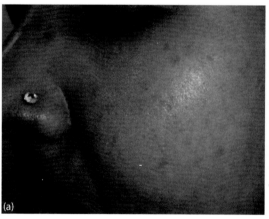
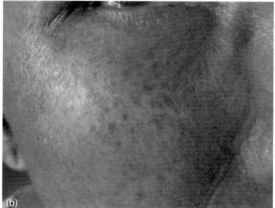

Figure 3.30 **(a, b)** Mat-like telangiectasia on cheek.

individuals. Other common body sites of distribution are palms (Figure 3.31), fingertips, and oral mucosa.[4] Sometimes the upper trunk is involved as well.

The presence of telangiectasia is indicative of ongoing vascular injury and systemic vasculopathy; the total number of telangiectasias in a given patient predicts the risk of pulmonary arterial hypertension.[3]

Pruritus

In progressive dSSc, there may be pruritus and pain during the edematous phase. Approximately 40% patients with dSSc may experience intense pruritus. The pain is characterized by the "pins and needles" sensation.[3]

Cutaneous features resulting from vasculopathy

RAYNAUD'S PHENOMENON

The most prominent vasculopathic manifestation in patients with SSc is Raynaud's phenomenon (RP). This may occur during the early stage and often may be the presenting feature. Body parts with end-vasculature, like distal fingers and toes are the most common sites of involvement. The tip

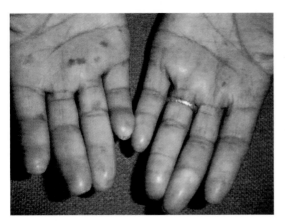

Figure 3.31 Telangiectasia of palms. Well-demarcated pallor of the finger-tips indicating associated Raynaud's phenomenon.

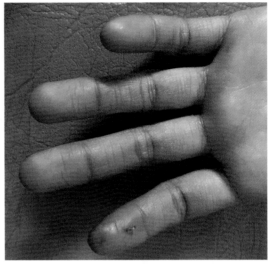

Figure 3.32 Bluish hue of the fingers and palm due to restoration of circulation in Raynaud's phenomenon.

of the nose and helices of the ears may sometimes be affected. Sudden exposure to cold water and lower environmental temperatures precipitate the episodes of RP. The other important triggering factor for RP in these patients is emotional stress.[3,4] The evolution of an episode of RP is through three phases of color changes (tri-color phenomenon).[3,4]

- Well-demarcated pallor (Figures 3.24 and 3.31) that may be painful (due to arterial vasospasm and ischemia)[4]
- Bluish/cyanotic hue (Figure 3.32), indicative of slow deoxygenated venous circulation
- Erythema (reactive hyperemia after circulation is re-established)

An acute episode subsides spontaneously or with the warming of the affected digits.

ULCERS

Digital small ulcers

Small, painful, superficial ulcers (Figure 3.33a and b) at the digital tips are frequent in patients with SSc and indicate ischemia of small terminal arteries and arterioles.[3,4] These heal with pitted (Figure 3.34)/stellate scars (Figure 3.35). Digital pitted scars are commonly encountered in these patients.

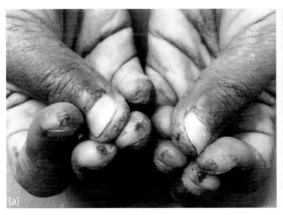

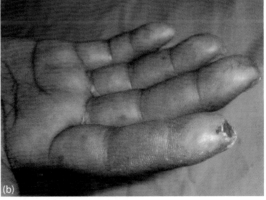

Figure 3.33 (a, b) Small superficial ulcers at the digital tips indicating ischemia of terminal arteries and arterioles.

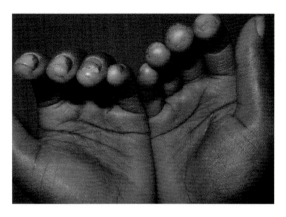

Figure 3.34 Pitted scars at digital tips.

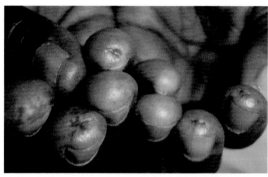

Figure 3.35 Digital ulcers healed with stellate scars.

Digital large ulcers

Larger, deeper, intensely painful ulcers (Figure 3.36a–c) may occur at distal digits due to occlusion of digital small arteries during an episode of vasospastic ischemia.[3,4] Larger tissue infarction (Figure 3.37), gangrene (Figure 3.38), and loss of the involved digit may occur secondary to larger arterial occlusion.[3,4]

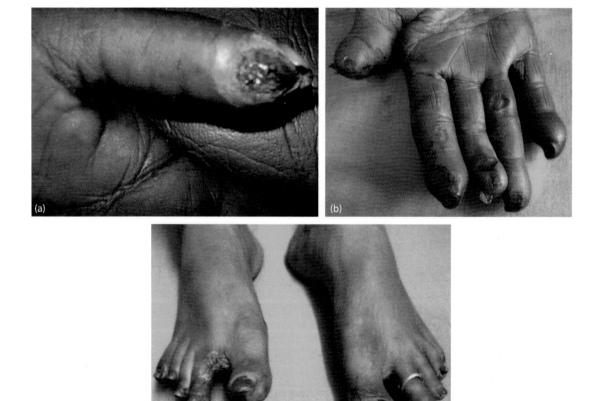

Figure 3.36 (a–c) Large, deep, painful ischemic ulcers at distal digits.

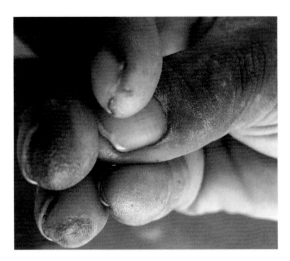

Figure 3.37 Digital tip infarctions.

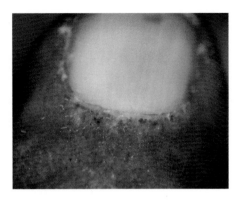

Figure 3.39 Dilated nail-fold capillaries visible without magnifying device.

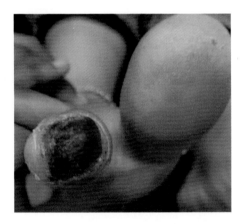

Figure 3.38 Gangrene of the toe in a patient with dSSc.

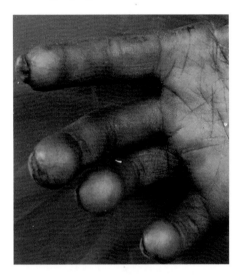

Figure 3.40 Hemispherical contour of the distal phalanges, the "Round finger pad sign."

NAILFOLD CAPILLARY CHANGES

Various patterns of nailfold capillary changes may occur in patients with PSS, clearly appreciated by videocapillaroscopy[7] or dermoscopy. However, often dilated capillaries are visible without magnifying devices (Figure 3.39).

SEQUELAE OF DIGITAL VASCULOPATHY

Digital vasculopathy causes a loss of soft tissue resulting in a flattening or rounded appearance of the distal pulp (Figure 3.40). This hemispheric contour of the digital tip is known as "round finger pad sign" or Mizutani's sign, frequently seen in ring fingers. The distal pulp may gradually be nearly lost (as illustrated in Figure 3.25).

Nail changes

With gradual attenuation of the distal pulp of the fingers and toes, the longitudinal diameter of the nails is reduced and a rectangular shape is attained (Figure 3.41). The hyponychium is obliterated as the tip of the pulp is adherent to the under surface of nail plate (Figure 3.42). This leads to an overhanging of the nail plate towards palmar aspect, giving a beaked appearance of the nails (Figure 3.43).

Calcinosis cutis

Calcinosis in patients with SSc occurs in a peri-articular location, mostly in clusters (Thieberge-Weissenbach syndrome).[3] These may present as

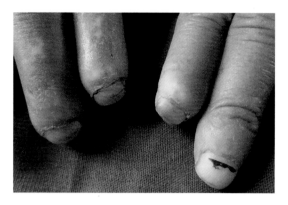

Figure 3.41 Rectangular shaped nails.

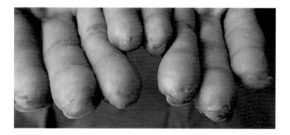

Figure 3.42 Tip of the pulp is adherent to the under surface of nail plate.

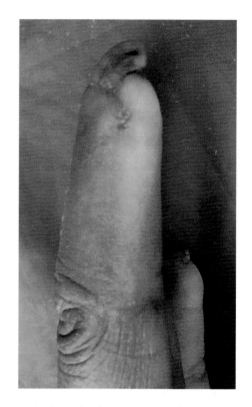

Figure 3.43 Beaked appearance of the nail.

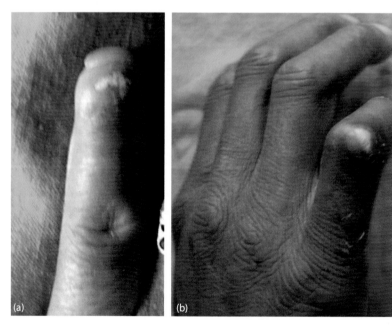

Figure 3.44 (a, b) Peri-articular calcinosis in a patient with dSSc.

acutely inflamed nodules around the joints, mimicking gout.[3] Later, the surface becomes white (Figure 3.44a and b). Over trauma-prone areas, the nodules may rupture through the skin with extrusion of thick, chalky material, termed as calcinosis cutis[3] (Figure 3.45).

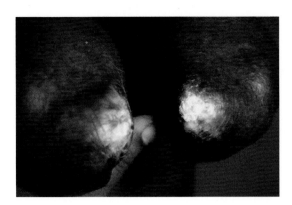

Figure 3.45 Calcinosis cutis.

SYSTEMIC MANIFESTATIONS

Musculoskeletal involvement

The musculoskeletal system is prominently involved in patients with PSS. Restriction of movements, joint pain, and the feelings of weakness experienced by these patients are of multifactorial origin. These include[3,4]:

- Sclerosis of the skin overlying the joints and peri-articular fibrosis
- Erosive polyarthritis specific for SSc
- Overlap of scleroderma and rheumatoid arthritis
- Disuse atrophy of muscles
- Extension of the fibrotic process to involve skeletal muscles in the background of severe cutaneous involvement in patients with dSSc (fibrosing myopathy).
- Associated inflammatory myopathy (5%–10%).
- Malnutrition (impaired food intake due to microstomia, dysphagia, and gastro-intestinal involvement related to the disease).

The details of musculoskeletal involvement have been presented in Table 3.1.[3,4]

Table 3.1 Musculoskeletal involvement in SSc

Involvement	Symptoms	Remarks
MCP, PIP, and DIP joints	Partial or total contracture in late fibrotic phase	Due to involvement of peri-articular soft tissues DIP joint involvement is rare.
Large joints: wrists, elbows, shoulders, hips, knees, ankles	Contracture	Initially due to fibrosis of the overlying skin, later fascia, joint capsule, and tendons are involved. Ankylosis of the joints is the sequelae.
Tendon friction rubs	Coarse crepitation over the large joints of extremities	Results from low-grade tenosynovitis, inflammatory edema, and fibrosis of the peri-articular tissue. Present in 15%–30% patients Common in dcSSc Indicates disease activity Poor prognostic indicator. Co-exists with severe vasculopathy, myopathy, renal involvement, and interstitial lung disease
Erosive polyarthritis		Relatively specific for SSc
Inflammatory muscle disease	Minimal to profound weakness of muscles of upper and lower extremities	Proximal > distal in 30% patients Poor disease outcome and increased morbidity
Fibrosing myopathy	Restricted joint mobility with muscle weakness	Cardiomyopathy, heart failure, and arrhythmias may be associated. These are severe and progressive.

Source: Boin, F., and Wigley, F.M., Clinical features and treatment of scleroderma, in: Firestein, G.S. et al. Eds., *Kelley's Textbook of Rheumatology*, 2, 9th ed., Elsevier Saunders, Philadelphia, PA, 1363–1403, 2015; Moinzadeh, P. et al., Scleroderma, in: Goldsmith, L.A. et al. Eds., *Fitzpatrick's Dermatology in General Medicine*, 2, 8th ed., McGraw-Hill Medical, New York, 1942–1956, 2012.

Gastro-intestinal involvement

Gastro-intestinal tract (GIT) is the most common viscera involved in SSc (80%).[2] The most frequent site of involvement in SSc is the esophagus. Various symptoms resulting from esophageal involvement have been presented in Table 3.2. Esophageal dysmotility and gastro-esophageal reflux are the most prominent symptoms.[2] There is a functional loss of the gastro-esophageal sphincter resulting in the hypotonia of the lower two-thirds of the esophagus. This may be a combined effect of neural and sphincteric smooth muscle involvement. In long-standing cases, complications may occur; these include esophageal ulcers, Barrett's esophagus, which may progress to adenocarcinoma, and peptic stricture/fistula formation.

Oropharyngeal involvement gives rise to difficulties in food intake (Box 3.1).[3,4] Various other symptoms related to gastro-intestinal involvement have been presented in Table 3.3.[3,4]

Gastric mucosa may be atrophic with loss of acid secretion resulting in indigestion. Various segments of the intestine are atonic and dilated, resulting in diverticula formation, segmental constrictions and pseudo-obstructions.[3,4] These may result from the combined effects of micro-vasculopathy, neural involvement, smooth muscle atrophy, and tissue fibrosis.[2] Asymptomatic, wide-mouthed diverticula are pathognomonic features of SSc.[3] Pneumatosis cystoides intestinalis may be an occasional finding. Extensive mucosal involvement results in malabsorption in these patients.

Pulmonary involvement

The two most frequent manifestations of pulmonary involvement are interstitial lung disease (ILD) and pulmonary arterial hypertension (PAH). ILD is the most common pulmonary involvement (80%) in patients with dSSc and is seen in 20% patients with lSSc.[2,3] PAH may occur both in lSSc

Table 3.2 Various symptoms due to esophageal involvement

Esophageal involvement	Symptomatology
Impaired peristalsis and dysmotility	• Difficulty in swallowing pills and solid foods, rather than liquids • Sense of sticking of food to the retro-sternal area • Retro-sternal pain (more at night)
Gastro-esophageal reflux	• Acid reflux causing esophagitis, resulting in heartburn • Stasis and regurgitation of food, especially in supine position • Nausea/vomiting

Source: Boin, F., and Wigley, F.M., Clinical features and treatment of scleroderma, in: Firestein, G.S. et al. Eds., *Kelley's Textbook of Rheumatology*, 2, 9th ed., Elsevier Saunders, Philadelphia, PA, 1363–1403, 2015; Moinzadeh, P. et al., Scleroderma, in: Goldsmith, L.A. et al. Eds., *Fitzpatrick's Dermatology in General Medicine*, 2, 8th ed., McGraw-Hill Medical, New York, 1942–1956, 2012.

BOX 3.1: Oropharyngeal involvement in patients with SSc affecting food intake[3,4]

Difficulty in food intake

• Reduced oral aperture hampering large bites, like biting an apple and inserting larger bolus of food to mouth

Difficulty in mastication

• Fibrosis and restricted mobility of facial skin and deeper tissue
• Tightening of perioral skin
• Loosening of teeth due to periodontal fibrosis and regression of gum
• Reduced salivary secretion

Difficulty in initiation of swallowing

• Upper pharyngeal myopathy in a subset of SSc patients
• Fibrosis of upper pharyngeal mucosa and esophagus

Risk of laryngeal aspiration

• Upper pharyngeal dysfunction causing food matters entering the laryngeal opening, resulting in recurrent cough during eating

Table 3.3 Gastro-intestinal involvement in patients with SSc

Involved part	Involvement	Symptoms
Stomach	Gastroparesis	• Early satiety • Gastro-esophageal reflux • Delayed gastric emptying (50%)[2] and bloating sensation • Gastritis and gastric ulceration
	Gastric mucosal atrophy	• Loss of gastric acid secretion and indigestion • Abdominal pain, nausea • Malabsorption
	Gastric antral vascular ectasia (GAVE): Abnormal angiogenesis leading to dilated micro-vessels and arterio-venous malformations.	• Occult gastric bleeding
Small & large intestine	Segments of atonic dilatation & constrictions resulting in dysmotility	• Alternate constipation and diarrhoea due to impaired peristalsis • Malabsorption, malnutrition and weight loss • Episodic pseudo-obstruction resulting in surgical emergencies • Rarely; volvulus, stricture, perforation

Source: Boin, F., and Wigley, F.M., Clinical features and treatment of scleroderma, in: Firestein, G.S. et al. Eds., *Kelley's Textbook of Rheumatology*, 2, 9th ed., Elsevier Saunders, Philadelphia, PA, 1363–1403, 2015; Moinzadeh, P. et al., Scleroderma, in: Goldsmith, L.A. et al. Eds., *Fitzpatrick's Dermatology in General Medicine*, 2, 8th ed., McGraw-Hill Medical, New York, 1942–1956, 2012.

and dSSc but it is typically associated with the former subset. ILD and PAH may co-exist in a given patient, but clinical manifestations of either of the one may predominate.[3] Pulmonary involvement in patients with SSc may be asymptomatic and progressive respiratory failure may be the presenting feature.

In the presence of ILD, bi-basilar fine inspiratory crepitations (Velcro rales) are the characteristic findings. Cough without expectoration develops at a later stage. Black, male patients with primary cardiac involvement have greater severity of ILD.[2]

PAH is present in 12% patients with SSc and is encountered in both the subsets of the disease.[2] The presenting features of PAH are dyspnea on exertion and fatigue. Progressive dyspnea, gradually leading to distress with minimal activity, tachycardia at rest, and cyanosis are the indicators of worsening PAH.[3,4] Occasionally, chest pain and syncope may be experienced.[3] PAH may remain asymptomatic for long duration (>10 years) and right heart failure may be the presenting feature.[3–5] Risk factors for development of ILD and PAH in patients with SSc have been presented in Table 3.4.[3]

Table 3.4 Risk factors for pulmonary involvement in patients with SSc

Interstitial lung disease	Pulmonary arterial hypertension
• dSSc • African-Americans & Native-Americans • Presence of anti-topoisomerase-1 antibody • Presence of anti-U3-RNP or anti-Th/To antibody	• Late-onset disease • lSSc • Presence of extensive telangiectasias • Presence of anticentromere antibody • Presence of anti-U3-RNP, anti-B23, anti-β_2 glycoprotein I antibodies • Low diffusing capacity (DLCO) in pulmonary function testing

Source: Boin, F., and Wigley, F.M., Clinical features and treatment of scleroderma, in: Firestein, G.S. et al. Eds., *Kelley's Textbook of Rheumatology*, 2, 9th ed., Elsevier Saunders, Philadelphia, PA, 1363–1403, 2015.

Pulmonary involvement is associated with high morbidity and approximately 60% deaths in patients with SSc.[2-4] PAH is the most frequent cause of SSc-related death.

Cardiac involvement

Prevalence of cardiac involvement in patients with SSc is variable between 10%–50%.[2,3] It may occur in both lSSc and dSSc. The cardinal feature of the primary cardiac involvement in SSc is focal myocardial fibrosis of the ventricles.[2,3] Heart failure, secondary to other organ involvement, may occur in the presence of ILD, PAH, or renal failure.[2,3]

Conduction defects and arrhythmias (endocardium), heart failure, valvular regurgitation (myocardium), and pericarditis/pericardial effusion (pericardium) are the cardiac manifestations of SSc.[2-5] Intramural coronary arterioles may be involved as part of myocardial fibrosis, resulting in vasospasm and reduced myocardial blood supply. Unlike in other collagen vascular disorders, atherosclerotic coronary artery disease is rare in SSc. The various factors determining reduced left-ventricular ejection fraction in these patients are[3]:

- Male gender
- Older age
- Presence of digital ulcers
- Myositis
- Non-use of calcium channel blockers

Cardiac involvement may not be manifest and remain unrecognized (75%).[2] Asymptomatic pericardial effusion may sometimes be recognized by echocardiography.[3] Electrocardiography often reveals arrhythmias and conduction abnormalities.[3]

BOX 3.2: Various causes of chest pain in patients with SSc[3-5]

- Musculoskeletal pain
- Esophageal reflux/dysmotility
- Pulmonary arterial hypertension
- Pericarditis/pericardial effusion
- Heart failure
- Cardiac arrhythmias

However, symptomatic cardiac manifestations are indicators of poor prognosis and reduced survival of patients with SSc.

Sudden onset chest pain in a patient with PSS may be multifactorial (Box 3.2), but a cardiac pain should never be missed.

Renal involvement

Clinically evident renal dysfunction is not as common in SSc as in other collagen vascular disorders. Mild renal involvement evidenced by proteinuria may be present in SSc. Scleroderma-renal crisis (SRC) is the most important renal involvement associated with this disorder. SRC is seen in 5%–10% of SSc patients.[3,4] It is usual in patients with dSSc and is rarely encountered in lSSc (1%–2%).[3,4] It is common to manifest by the initial four years of the disease onset [3,4] but rare in the later stages of disease. A variable combination of sudden-onset, severe hypertension, sudden renal failure, and microangiopathic hemolytic anemia in a patient with SSc should rouse the possibility of SRC.[3,4] The clinical and laboratory indicators of SRC are presented in Table 3.5.

Table 3.5 Clinical and laboratory indicators of SRC

Clinical	Laboratory
1. Abrupt onset of very high blood pressure (>150/90 mmHg)	1. High/rapid rise of serum creatinine
2. Dyspnoea (pulmonary edema/congestive cardiac failure)	2. Proteinuria ±, microscopic hematuria, granular casts (these parameters may be normal)
3. Acute/sub-acute onset of: confusion, lethargy, fatigue, headache, altered vision (encephalopathy)	3. Hemolytic anemia/thrombocytopenia
4. Sudden blindness (hypertensive retinopathy)	4. Raised plasma renin

Source: Boin, F., and Wigley, F.M., Clinical features and treatment of scleroderma, in: Firestein, G.S. et al. Eds., *Kelley's Textbook of Rheumatology*, 2, 9th ed., Elsevier Saunders, Philadelphia, PA, 1363–1403, 2015.

BOX 3.3: Various risk factors for development of SRC[3]

- Diffuse cutaneous disease, with rapidly progressive sclerosis
- Patients with dSSc, treated with high dose systemic corticosteroids (>40 mg prednisolone/day)/long term low-dose prednisolone (>15 mg/day)
- Low-dose cyclosporine
- African-American races
- ANA positivity (speckled pattern), anti-U3-RNP positivity

The clinical features showing association with SRC are large joint contractures and high initial modified Rodnan Score (>20).[8]

Various risk factors for the development of SRC in these disorders are presented in Box 3.3.[3] Male gender and serum creatinine level >3 mg/mL are the poor prognostic factors in presence of SRC.[3]

MORBIDITY ASSOCIATED WITH SSc

The principal cause of morbidity in patients with SSc is the gross change in physical appearance, resulting in great psychological stress and depression.[2] There is restricted mobility because of contracted joints and dyspnea from pulmonary involvement. Functional restriction occurs due to painful RP and digital ulcers. All these hamper day-to-day activities to the extent that the patients may need constant aid from others. Difficulty in food intake results in significant nutritional deficiency. Sexual function is impaired in both the genders; this is more affected in male patients who may develop erectile dysfunction due to microvasculopathy.[2] Overall, the quality of life is greatly jeopardized in these patients.

DISEASE COURSE AND COMPLICATIONS

The clinical course of SSc is chronic and progressive without evidence of sudden flares, classically described as the "monophasic course." The life-threatening complications of SSc include PAH and SRC.

In various studies, the predictors of a reduced survival and increased mortality in patients with SSc are renal and cardio-pulmonary involvement,[1,9] male gender, gastrointestinal involvement,[9] and investigative findings such as low diffusion lung capacity with carbon monoxide (DLCO), proteinuria, raised erythrocyte sedimentation rate (ESR),[10] and autoantibody profile like the presence of anti-topoisomerase-1[1] and absence of anti-centromere antibody (ACA).[1,8]

ILD and PAH are the major causes of death in patients with SSc. PAH usually develops late in the disease, beyond 10 years of initial disease manifestation and carries significant risk of mortality. Patients with lSSc are more likely to develop morbidity and mortality related to PAH. A UK nationwide registry (2009) reported survival rates of SSc-related PAH at the first and third years were 78%–47%, respectively. High right atrial pressure at diagnosis, higher mean pulmonary artery pressure, and low cardiac index are the predictors of higher mortality.[11] Co-existent ILD and PAH carries a poor prognostic factor, with a three-year survival of 39%.[2,12] Currently, PAH is the most common cause of SSc-related death (60%).

Mortality associated with SRC is high with a five-year survival rate of 59%.[2,13] The poor prognostic factors include male gender, age >53 years, normotensive patients at presentation, and long-term need for dialysis. Patients with heart failure and initial serum creatinine level >265 µmol/L may require life-long dialysis. The majority of the patients with SRC may require dialysis, but normal renal function may be resumed in some within six months.[3]

Significant cardiac involvement giving rise to hemodynamic instability may occur in 10% patients.[2,14] An estimated 4.5% death in patients with SSc is due to cardiac involvement.[2] Age, male gender, digital ulcers, myositis, and pulmonary disease were the independent associations of LV dysfunctions in the EUSTAR database.[15] Echocardiographic evidence of right ventricular dysfunction and a higher New York Heart Association (NYHA) functional class are associated with poor prognosis.[3]

Gastrointestinal involvement may have a mortality of 6%–12%.[2]

Patients with SSc are susceptible to develop various malignancies and related risk of mortality. These include esophageal and oropharyngeal carcinomas, hepatocellular carcinoma, hematopoietic malignancies, and lung and skin cancers.[2]

Currently, pulmonary involvement is the leading cause of death in patients with SSc, followed by SRC. However, with the use of a specific vasodilator therapy for pulmonary involvement and early institution of ACE-inhibitors as renoprotective agents, the survival rate of patients with SSc has improved as compared to earlier.[2] Children with SSc have a better survival as compared to adults.[2]

REFERENCES

1. Ioannidis JP, Vlachoyiannopoulos PG, Haidich AB et al. Mortality in systemic sclerosis: An international meta-analysis of individual patient data. *Am J Med* 2005;118:2–10.
2. Nikpour M, Stevens WM, Herrick AL, Proudman SM. Epidemiology of systemic sclerosis. *Best Pract Res Clin Rheumatol* 2010;24:857–869.
3. Boin F, Wigley FM. Clinical features and treatment of scleroderma. In: Firestein GS, Budd RC, Gabriel SE, McInnes IB, O'Dell JR, Eds. *Kelley's Textbook of Rheumatology*, Vol. 2, 9th ed. Philadelphia, PA: Elsevier Saunders, 2013, pp. 1363–1403.
4. Moinzadeh P, Denton CP, Krieg T, Black CM. Scleroderma. In: Goldsmith LA, Katz SI, Gilchrest BA, Paller AS, Leffell DJ, Wolff K, Eds. *Fitzpatrick's Dermatology in General Medicine*, Vol 2, 8th ed. New York: McGraw-Hill Medical, 2012, pp. 1942–1956.
5. Orteu CH, Denton CP. Systemic sclerosis. In: Griffiths CEM, Barker J, Bleiker T, Chalmers R, Creamer D, Eds. *Rook's Textbook of Dermatology*, Vol 2, 9th ed. Oxford, UK: Wiley Blackwell, 2016, pp. 56.1–56.23.
6. Ritchie B. Pulmonary function in scleroderma. *Thorax* 1964;19:28–36.
7. Herrick AL, Clark S. Quantifying digital vascular disease in patients with primary Raynaud's phenomenon and systemic sclerosis. *Ann Rheum Dis* 1998;57:70–78.
8. DeMarco PJ, Weisman MH, Seibold JR et al. Predictors and outcomes of scleroderma renal crisis: The high-dose versus low-dose D penicillamine in early diffuse systemic sclerosis trial. *Arthritis Rheum* 2002;46:2983–2989.
9. Mayes MD, Lacey JVJ, Beebe-Dimmer J et al. Prevalence, incidence, survival, and disease characteristics of systemic sclerosis in a large US population. *Arthritis Rheum* 2003;48:2246–2255.
10. Assassi S, Del Junco D, Sutter K et al. Clinical and genetic factors predictive of mortality in early systemic sclerosis. *Arthritis Rheum* 2009;61:1403–1411.
11. Bryan C, Knight C, Black CM, Silman AJ. Prediction of five-year survival following presentation with scleroderma: Development of a simple model using disease factors at first visit. *Arthritis Rheum* 1999;42:2660–2665.
12. Mathai SC, Hummers LK, Champion HC et al. Survival in pulmonary hypertension associated with the scleroderma spectrum of diseases: Impact of interstitial lung disease. *Arthritis Rheum* 2009;60:569–577.
13. Penn H, Howie AJ, Kingdon EJ et al. Scleroderma renal crisis: Patient characteristics and long-term outcomes. *Q J Med* 2007;100:485–494.
14. Domsic R, Fasanella K, Bielefeldt K. Gastrointestinal manifestations of systemic sclerosis. *Dig Dis Sci* 2008;53:1163–1174.
15. Allanore Y, Meune C, Vonk MC et al. Prevalence and factors associated with left ventricular dysfunction in the EULAR Scleroderma Trial and Research Group (EUSTAR) database of patients with systemic sclerosis. *Ann Rheum Dis* 2010;69:218–221.

4

Investigations and diagnosis

ARUN C. INAMADAR AND AJIT B. JANAGOND

INTRODUCTION

Diagnosis of systemic sclerosis (SSc) is mostly clinical. Constellation of clinical features like, Raynaud's phenomenon, sclerodactyly, digital ulcers, gradual evolution to widespread cutaneous sclerosis, and specific systemic involvement are the characteristics of the disorder. The EULAR/ACR classification criteria is the most recent method for diagnosis of SSc.[1] This score-based diagnostic tool is helpful in the confirmation of even the early cases under evolution, with limited disease at presentation and exclusion of various conditions which may mimic SSc.[1,2]

The individual criterion utilized in the EULAR/ACR classification system[1] is mostly clinical. However, demonstration of scleroderma-specific autoantibodies, nailfold capillaries, and confirmation of pulmonary involvement call for various diagnostic assistance.

The laboratory parameters, immunological investigations, and imaging techniques helpful in supporting the diagnosis of SSc have been described in the following section. Some of these are very useful methods in predicting the disease course and individual patient outcome.[3] Symptom-based investigation protocol may miss early features of pulmonary and cardiac involvement. Hence, baseline and follow-up screening for organ involvement should always be included in the management strategy of these patients.

LABORATORY INVESTIGATIONS

Complete blood count with erythrocyte sedimentation rate (ESR) should be undertaken at presentation. This helps in the assessment of the baseline hematological parameters of individual patients as well as establishes a work-up for subsequent immunosuppressive therapy.[3] Normocytic, normochromic anemia of chronic disease, is expected in these patients. Microcytic, hypochromic anemia, may be present in the presence of nutritional deficiency, which is common in these patients.

Thrombocytopenia and evidence of hemolytic anemia may be associated with scleroderma renal crisis (SRC).[3,4]

Baseline blood urea nitrogen and creatinine levels are to be estimated in all patients. High serum creatinine at any point of the disease course or rapid increase in serum creatinine level in association with malignant hypertension is the indicator of SRC.[3,4]

Urine microscopy and urinary protein estimation should be done at initial visit. If proteinuria is present, urinary protein excretion in 24 hours has to be quantified. The presence of microscopic hematuria and granular casts, with or without proteinuria, is one of the laboratory indicators of SRC.[3,4]

AUTOANTIBODIES

The three main categories of SSc-specific autoantibodies in these patients are the anti-centromere antibodies, antitopoisomerase-I, and anti-RNA polymerase III.[2-4] These antibodies predict the clinical pattern of skin involvement, organ involvement, disease evolution, complications, and overall prognosis in an individual patient (Table 4.1).[2,4] Using Hep-2 cells as a substrate, the centromere staining pattern is observed in the CREST syndrome; fine and coarse speckled pattern and a ground-glass appearance is seen in the presence of the Scl-70 antibody.[5]

Antibodies to PM/Scl and U1-RNP are associated with scleroderma overlap syndromes; anti-PM/Scl with myositis, pulmonary fibrosis, and acro-osteolysis

Table 4.1 Antibody-specific clinical characteristics, risk factors, and disease course in patients with scleroderma

Anti-centromere antibodies (ACA)	Anti-topoisomerase-1 (Scl-70) (ATA)	Anti-RNA polymerase III (ARA/RNAP)
• Older, white women • Limited cutaneous disease: features of CREST are frequent • Severe Raynaud's phenomenon • Risk of digital ulcer • Risk for macrovascular disease; frequent digital gangrene and amputation • Subcutaneous calcinosis • ILD less frequent • PAH and right heart failure more common • Indolent course; delayed diagnosis • Prognosis: comparatively favorable	• African-American patients • Diffuse cutaneous disease: rapid evolution and severe skin involvement (1–3 years) • Risk of digital ulcer • Raynaud's phenomenon may be the first symptom • Joint and tendon involvement leading to contracted fingers and elbows are frequent • ILD is strongly associated, but not indicative of disease severity • At risk of SRC • Prognosis: Poor. Associated with high mortality	• Diffuse cutaneous disease: most severe skin involvement with rapid and widespread progression • Involvement of subcutaneous tissue, muscles, tendon, and underlying joints is frequent. Joint flexion contractures may occur by few months of disease onset • Tendon friction rub frequent • At risk of fibrosing myopathy • Usually negative in patients with digital ulcer • Severe gastrointestinal involvement • Relatively less pulmonary involvement (ILD & PAH) • High risk of SRC (25%–40%) at early phase of rapid skin change

Source: van den Hoogen, F. et al., *Ann. Rheum. Dis.*, 72, 1747–1755, 2013; Boin, F., and Wigley, F.M., Clinical features and treatment of scleroderma, in: Firestein, G.S. et al. Eds., *Kelley's Textbook of Rheumatology*, vol. 2, 9th ed., Elsevier Saunders, Philadelphia, PA, 1363–1403, 2013; Nikpour, M. et al., *Best Pract. Res. Clin. Rheumatol.*, 24, 857–869, 2010.

Abbreviations: CREST: Calcinosis, Raynaud's phenomenon, Esophageal dysmotility, Sclerodactyly, Telangiectasia, ILD: Interstitial lung disease, PAH: Pulmonary arterial hypertension, SRC: Scleroderma renal crisis.

Table 4.2 Frequency of various autoantibodies in disease subsets of SSc

Autoantibodies	dSSc	lSSc	SSc-overlap syndromes
Anti-centromere antibodies	30%	10%	
Anti-topoisomerase-1 (Scl-70)	5%–7%	50%	
Anti-RNA polymerase III	25%	2%	
Anti-U1-RNP	15% (lSSc >> dSSc)		SSc-SLE (44%)
Anti-PM-Scl (polymyositis-scleroderma)	5% (dSSc > lSSc)		SSc-Myositis (33%)
Anti-U3-RNP (Anti-fibrillarin)	5%		
Anti-Ku	2%		
Anti-U11/U12 RNP	3%		
Th/To		5%	

Source: van den Hoogen, F. et al., Ann. Rheum. Dis., 72, 1747–1755, 2013.
Abbreviations: PM-Scl: Polymyositis-scleroderma, RNP: Ribonucleoprotein.

and anti-U1-RNP with systemic lupus erythematosus, inflammatory arthritis, and pulmonary fibrosis.[4]

The frequency of various autoantibodies in the subsets of the disease, dSSc, lSSc, and scleroderma overlap syndromes has been presented in Table 4.2.[1]

ORGAN-SPECIFIC INVESTIGATIONS

Assessment of skin fibrosis

The degree of skin fibrosis can be assessed clinically as well as by other measures. The modified Rodnan skin score (mRSS) is the clinical method to assess the extent of skin involvement.[4,6] A trained clinician assesses the skin thickness at 17 different body areas as mentioned in Table 4.3.

A high mRSS score during baseline disease evaluation carries a poor prognosis of the disease (dSSc)[1] and is considered as a surrogate marker of overall disease severity.[7]

Other techniques for assessment of skin thickening are[3,4,8]:

- Ultrasound (20-MHz)
- Magnetic Resonance Imaging (MRI)
- Optical coherence tomography: provides a high contrast image of skin illustrating a decrease in optical density of the upper dermis; this finding corroborates with mRSS and histopathological evidence of dermal fibrosis
- Physical procedures (Plicometer, Durometer, Cutometer, Elastometer)

Table 4.3 Body sites for evaluation of skin fibrosis in mRSS

Body site	Maximum score	Subtotal score	Total score
Face	3	9	51
Thorax	3		
Abdomen	3		
Upper arm (right & left)	3 + 3	42	
Forearm (right & left)	3 + 3		
Hand (right & left)	3 + 3		
Fingers (right & left)	3 + 3		
Thighs (right & left)	3 + 3		
Legs (right & left)	3 + 3		
Feet (right & left)	3 + 3		

0 = No sclerosis, 1 = Mild skin sclerosis, 2 = Moderate skin sclerosis, 3 = Severe skin sclerosis.
Source: Orteu, C.H., and Denton, C.P., Systemic sclerosis, in: Griffiths, C. et al. Eds., Rook's Textbook of Dermatology, vol. 2, 9th ed., Wiley Blackwell, Oxford, UK, 56.1–56.23, 2016; Boin, F., and Wigley, F.M., Clinical features and treatment of scleroderma, in: Firestein, G.S. et al. Eds., Kelley's Textbook of Rheumatology, vol. 2, 9th ed., Elsevier Saunders, Philadelphia, PA, 1363–1403, 2013.

Histopathology

Skin biopsy and histopathological examination is not an absolute requirement in the diagnostic algorithm of SSc. However, histopathological features of SSc are characteristic and helpful in differentiating from other scleroderma-like conditions.

In the early inflammatory stage of the disease, there is a mild inflammatory infiltrate around the dermal blood vessels, cutaneous appendages, and the subcutaneous fat.[9] The dermal collagen may appear swollen at this stage. In the late sclerotic stage of the disease, the epidermis may be atrophic with a flattening of the rete ridges (Figure 4.1). The dermal collagen characteristics are altered; it appears homogenous and densely eosinophilic at lower magnification.[2,9] At higher power, the collagen bundles are closely packed and horizontally oriented parallel to the skin surface[2,9] (Figure 4.2).

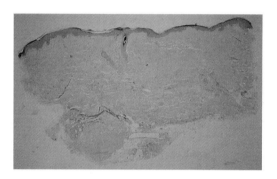

Figure 4.1 Epidermis is thinned out with a flattening of the rete ridges. Also note the square shape of the tissue block rather than the usual triangular shape, indicating tissue fibrosis (H&E stain, 4×).

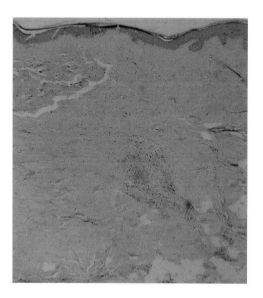

Figure 4.2 Homogenization of collagen is seen in the dermis (H&E stain, 10×).

There is evidence of fibrosis in the form of obliteration of appendages (hair follicles, sweat glands), which appear chinked and pulled up in the papillary dermis.[2,9] The dermal vessels are sparse with a thickening and hyalinization of the vessel walls and narrowing of the lumen. Aggregates of calcium may be present in sclerotic, homogenous collagen.

Assessment of cutaneous microcirculation

PROVOCATION TEST TO ELICIT RAYNAUD'S PHENOMENON

Raynaud's phenomenon (RP) may be florid, acute episodes being precipitated by lower environmental temperature and emotional stress. In patients with subtle features of RP, or in situations where adequate clinical history suggestive of RP are not available, provocation tests may be undertaken to induce RP.[10]

Cold-challenge test

The patient's fingers are dipped in a basin of cold water (10°C) for five minutes, and the clinical signs for RP are looked for.[11] Following immersion in cold water, the presence of RP can be substantiated by various techniques; high frequency ultrasound has been used for direct imaging of the digital arteries and the level of arterial closure assessed as a mean decrease in digital artery diameter expressed as a percentage of original diameter.[12] Inflatable tourniquet can be used around a finger for five minutes to assess cold-induced ischemia and post-ischemic reactive hyperaemia following its removal; it is compared to an adjacent finger taken as control.[12]

Infrared thermography

Infrared thermography is a technique to provide a pictorial representation of skin surface temperature, which is an indirect evidence of blood flow through the area. In doubtful cases, it is a useful tool to elicit evidence of RP. The hands of the patient are immersed in cold water (15°C) for one minute, and following 10 minutes the fingertip re-warming is recorded using infrared thermogram as compared to normal hands.[2] Use of this technique is restricted to specialized centres only.[2]

Finger systolic blood pressure measurement

Finger systolic blood pressure measurement in patients with RP demonstrates a marked reduction in systolic BP in response to cooling of the limb when compared to control.[8]

However, such tests may be cumbersome to be conducted at bed-side. Simple dipping of the fingers in cold water (below room temperature) may elicit initial pallor followed by bluish discoloration, suggestive of RP (Figure 4.3).

LASER DOPPLER FLOW MONITORING

Laser Doppler flow monitoring is a well-established method to assess the cutaneous microcirculation. However, its use is limited by wide signal variation from site to site and with positioning and orientation of the probe.[8]

Other such techniques include Doppler ultrasound and plethysmography.[8]

Demonstration of nailfold capillary pattern

Demonstration of nailfold capillary pattern is important in differentiating scleroderma-associated RP from primary Raynaud's disease and helps in disease categorization (lSSc/dSSc).[2,4]

The simple earlier technique to visualize nailfold capillaries is putting immersion oil at nailfolds and visualizing the area with bifocal dissecting

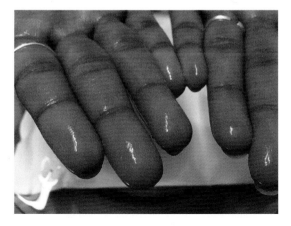

Figure 4.3 Bluish discoloration of the fingers following immersion in cold water in a patient of SSc without overt RP.

microscope or handheld ophthalmoscope (20–40 dioptres).[2] Computerised video-capillaroscopy is the standard technique for illustration of nailfold capillaries in patients with SSc.[2]

The normal architecture of nailfold capillaries is thin, palisading loops of blood vessels.[2,13] Using video-capillaroscopy at room temperature of 20°C–22°C, three patterns of nailfold capillary changes have been described in patients with SSc.[2] Changes in capillary density and architecture are studied and categorization is done according to disease duration and activity (Table 4.4).[2,13]

Nailfold video-capillaroscopic findings may be the early manifestation of scleroderma-associated microangiopathy and may precede major organ involvement.[8] Moreover, these changes may indicate the evolution of microangiopathy in a given patient and help in longitudinal follow up of the patients.[8] Demonstration of late pattern at presentation indicates disease of longer duration.[2]

Table 4.4 Nailfold video-capillaroscopic pattern in patients with SSc

Pattern	Findings
Early	Well-preserved capillary architecture and density
	Few enlarged/giant capillaries
	Few areas of hemorrhage
	No evident loss of capillaries
Active	Moderate loss of capillary density
	Mild disorganization of capillary architecture
	Frequent dilated/giant/tortuous capillary loops
	Frequent areas of micro-hemorrhage
	Rare ramified capillaries
Late	Severe disorganization of normal capillary architecture
	Severe loss of capillaries (dropout)
	Extensive avascular areas
	Very few giant capillaries and absence of hemorrhage
	Ramified/bushy capillaries (indicates neovascularization)

Source: Orteu, C.H., and Denton, C.P., Systemic sclerosis, in: Griffiths, C. et al. Eds., *Rook's Textbook of Dermatology*, vol. 2, 9th ed., Wiley Blackwell, Oxford, UK, 56.1–56.23, 2016; Cutolo, M. et al., *Rheumatology*, 43, 719–726, 2004.

RP may be the initial presentation of SSc, when other classical cutaneous or systemic features are not clinically evident. Differentiation from primary RP at this stage is an important step in the early diagnosis; demonstration of nailfold capillary changes is an important parameter towards confirmation of diagnosis of SSc.[2,8] Patients with RP and nailfold capillary abnormalities may develop clinical features of SSc (20%–30% cases) by the next 2–3 years.[8] Presence of scleroderma-specific autoantibodies, in addition to the above two features, increases the possibility of future development of SSc (70%–80%).[8]

At present, a dermoscope is widely used for the visualization of nailfold capillary changes with comparable accuracy (Figure 4.4a and b).[2]

Assessment of musculoskeletal system

In the presence of muscle weakness, a full range of investigations to establish inflammatory muscle disease must be performed. Estimation of muscle enzymes, electromyography, and magnetic resonance imaging (MRI) guided biopsy of individual group of muscles are helpful.[4]

Joint function is mostly assessed clinically by visible joint contracture, degree of limitation of movement, and tendon/bursa friction rubs.[7] Of these, the latter indicates disease activity, whereas the former two are indicators of end-stage articular and periarticular tissue involvement.[7] Finger joints have been considered as the representative for functional assessment as these are almost universally involved.[7] The "hand spread" and the "finger to palm distance in flexion (FTP)" techniques are in use for this purpose.[7] The third fingertip and distal palmar crease distance are measured in FTP; value of 0–0.09 cm is considered normal and 5.0+ cm is considered as the end-stage disease.[7] However, application of these techniques are difficult in already contracted finger joints and have not been standardized. The hand-mobility in scleroderma (HAMIS) test[14] and Duruoz hand index (DHI)[15] are the other measures to assess joint function in patients with scleroderma.

Investigations for pulmonary involvement

Patients with SSc require repeated pulmonary screening for interstitial lung disease (ILD) and pulmonary arterial hypertension (PAH). Parenchymal and vascular involvement, either alone or in combination, contributes to significant disease morbidity.[2–4,8] End-stage pulmonary disease contributes to death in approximately 60% patients with SSc and has been considered as the major cause of mortality.[4,8]

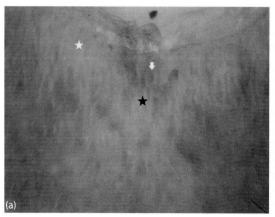
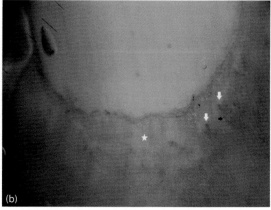

Figure 4.4 (a) Dermoscopy of the nailfold capillaries in SSc: Many avascular areas (black star) and disorganization of the vascular architecture (yellow star); bushy capillaries are indicated by yellow arrow. (b) Dermoscopy of the nailfold capillaries in SSc: Loss of normal capillary architecture. Dilated capillary loops (yellow arrows), giant capillaries (black arrow), and avascular areas (yellow star) are noted. (Courtesy of Dr. B.S. Ankad, S.N. Medical College, Bagalkot, Karnataka India.)

PULMONARY FUNCTION TEST

The pulmonary function test (PFT) is the gold-standard method to detect the lungs' involvement at an early stage. Abnormal PFT has been encountered in 70% patients with SSc.[8] Decrease in single breath "diffusion capacity using carbon monoxide (DLCO)" is a predictor of pulmonary vascular compromise.[4,8] The gradual fall in DLCO correlates with the severity of PAH and worse disease prognosis.[4,8] A value ≤75% is considered as an early marker of co-existent ILD and PAH.[4,8] However, declining DLCO is not specific of ILD and may be found in other pulmonary disease unrelated to SSc.[4]

Most specific components of PFT in diagnosis and follow-up of patients of SSc with restrictive lung disease (ILD) are forced vital capacity (FVC) and total lung capacity (TLC).[4,8] In all patients with SSc, PFT must be estimated at baseline; a normal value at baseline should be re-evaluated at 4–6 months intervals for early detection of impairment.[4,8] Thereafter, yearly estimation is recommended as severe ILD may develop by the third year of disease onset.[4,8]

A >10% fall in baseline FVC indicates progressive disease activity and warrants higher mortality in a given patient.[4] However, in some patients, the ILD may stabilize after the initial few months of onset as indicated by no further decline in follow up FVC values.[4]

CHEST RADIOGRAPH

Shrinking lung volume due to parenchymal fibrosis and bi-basilar reticular interstitial thickening are the features of ILD[4,8] (Figure 4.5). Honeycombing of the lungs parenchyma and bronchiectasis may be evident.[4,8] Spontaneous pneumothorax may be seen rarely. However, early stage ILD may be suspected clinically and is not detectable by chest X-Ray. Any patient of SSc suffering from sudden-onset cough, with or without expectoration, must be screened with a chest X-ray to rule out pneumonia (Figure 4.6); even aspiration pneumonia is common in these patients in presence of regurgitation.

HIGH RESOLUTION COMPUTED TOMOGRAPHY SCAN (HRCT)

HRCT is at par with PFT for detection of ILD in patients with SSc.[4,8] A patient with abnormal PFT

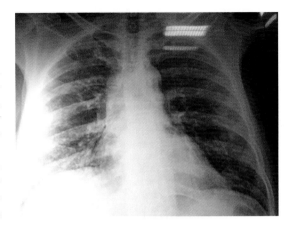

Figure 4.5 Chest X-ray (PA view): Multiple reticulonodular opacities noted in bilateral lung fields more in the right-lower zone, suggestive of interstitial lung disease.

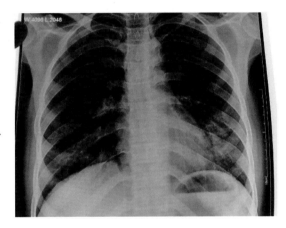

Figure 4.6 Consolidation of the left-lower lobe, suggestive of pneumonia in a patient with dSSc.

almost always displays pulmonary fibrosis in HRCT.[4,8] Findings observed at the various stages of development of ILD have been presented in Table 4.5 (see also Figure 4.7).

HRCT is more sensitive than a chest X-ray in detecting diffuse pulmonary involvement.[4,8] Close correlation of HRCT findings with PFT makes the combination of both the modalities a good predictor of disease prognosis.[4,8] FVC <70% or disease extent in HRCT >20% is the predictor of high mortality.[4,8] A staging system for determining prognosis of SSc patients with ILD using FVC and HRCT has been proposed.[16] This combined technique categorizes SSc-related ILD as

Table 4.5 HRCT findings in various stages of ILD in patients with SSc

Stage of ILD	HRCT findings
Early changes	Sub-pleural linear opacities in lung parenchyma in the posterior and basilar portions without alteration of the architecture
Advanced disease	Initially "ground-glass" opacities Later, fine, reticular opacities
Pulmonary fibrosis	Parenchymal distortion, reticular, intralobular, interstitial thickening, traction bronchiectasis, and bronchiolectasis The above is followed by honeycomb appearance and cystic air spaces (Figure 4.7)

Source: Boin, F., and Wigley, F.M., Clinical features and treatment of scleroderma, in: Firestein, G.S. et al. Eds., *Kelley's Textbook of Rheumatology*, vol. 2, 9th ed., Elsevier Saunders, Philadelphia, PA, 1363–1403, 2013; Nikpour, M. et al., *Best Pract. Res. Clin. Rheumatol.*, 24, 857–869, 2010.

a "limited" or "extensive" disease and is easily applicable in both clinical practice and research purpose.

The presence of PAH is confirmed by right heart catheterization, which, though invasive, is considered as the gold-standard technique.[4,8] Mean pulmonary arterial pressure ≥25 mm Hg at rest and pulmonary capillary wedge pressure ≤15 mm Hg as determined by right heart catheterization are indicative of PAH.[4,8] The DETECT algorithm is an evidence-based, non-invasive way to diagnose PAH at an early stage, or in patients with minimal symptoms.[17]

Investigations for cardiac involvement

Primary cardiac abnormalities are relatively unusual as compared to secondary involvement due to PAH. Electrocardiography (ECG) is useful in detecting cardiac arrhythmias, conduction defects, and pericardial effusion encountered in these patients.[4,7,8] In the early stage of PAH, an ECG may be normal. In advanced PAH, features of right ventricular hypertrophy and right axis deviation are evident.[4,8] The Holter monitor test can be performed to detect occult arrhythmias.[7]

Echocardiography is useful in detecting left ventricular dysfunction resulting from myocardial fibrosis, pericarditis, and pericardial effusion.[7] Transthoracic Doppler echocardiography may be done to detect right ventricular diastolic dysfunction, restricted ejection fraction, valvular insufficiency, inter-ventricular septal dysmotility, valvular regurgitation, and other functional abnormalities.[4,8] Tricuspid annular plane systolic excursion (TAPSE) of <1.8 cm in a patient with PAH is indicative of high mortality.[4]

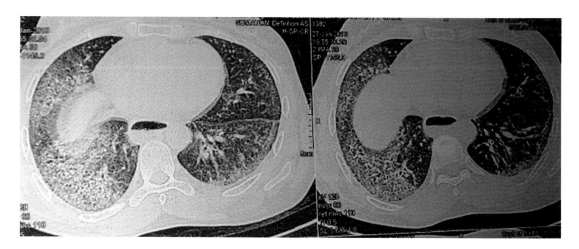

Figure 4.7 HRCT of thorax: Architectural distortion of the lung fields; bilateral reticulo-nodular opacities are noted in the sub-pleural location (more on the right posterior aspect). Multiple cysts are noted in the right basal segments giving rise to "honeycomb appearance." Thickening of the septa and bilateral oblique fissures noted.

Increased right ventricular systolic pressure (RVSP) is a useful indicator of PAH.[4,8] Estimation of plasma N-terminal pro-B-type natriuretic peptide BNP (NT-proBNP) helps in detecting right or left heart strain, and an elevated level is an indirect indicator of PAH.[4,8] This may also indicate primary cardiac involvement.[7] Higher mortality is associated with a high (10-fold rise) level of NT-proBNP.[3]

Subclinical cardiac involvement may be detected by Thallium-201 single photon emission computed tomographic scan (SPECT), cardiac MRI, or echocardiography.[7]

The overall cardiopulmonary status of a patient with SSc may be assessed by a "6-minute walk distance"[7]; however, interpretation of the test may be difficult because of restricted mobility in these patients resulting from musculoskeletal involvement.[7]

Investigations for renal involvement

SRC is the dreaded renal complication in patients with SSc and was earlier considered as the most common cause of mortality in these patients. History of SRC is considered as the determinant for presence or absence of renal involvement. Serum creatinine and creatinine clearance are the parameters to be monitored for grading of renal involvement in patients with history of SRC. Based on these, the severity of renal involvement has been graded as mild, moderate, severe, and end-stage (grades 1–4).[7] Mild renal involvement is considered with a history of SRC, serum creatinine level <1.5 mg/dL, and creatinine clearance >100 cc/minute; end-stage renal disease is considered with the patient requiring dialysis, serum creatinine ≥5 mg/dL, and creatinine clearance <30 cc/minute.[7]

Investigations for gastro-intestinal tract involvement

Any patient with SSc must be thoroughly screened for gastro-intestinal involvement, even in absence of overt symptoms. This is because such symptoms may be subjective and may not be true indicator of the underlying involvement.

Upper GI endoscopy is indicated to look for esophagitis, strictures, bleeding, and Barrett's esophagus.[3,4,8] Some patients may require periodic upper GI endoscopy to rule out gradual development of esophageal malignancy.[3,8] The gastric antral vascular ectasia (GAVE) can be diagnosed by

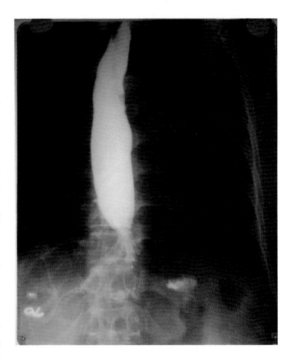

Figure 4.8 Barium swallow study of the esophagus showing dilatation of the middle and lower segments.

endoscopy as longitudinal convergent red strips of vasculature at the pylorus (watermelon stomach).[4,8]

Esophageal motility can be detected by several methods. A barium-swallow radiography may detect an atonic dilated esophagus[7] (Figure 4.8). Other modern techniques include cine-esophagography, 24-hours pH-manometry, and esophageal scintigraphy following radio labeled meal.[3]

DIAGNOSIS

The classification criteria for SSc has undergone repeated modifications over the years. In absence of any hallmark diagnostic test for the condition, several sets of diagnostic criteria have been developed to prove or rule out the diagnosis of SSc.[1] These classification criteria include clinical and diagnostic parameters necessary for the diagnosis of SSc; moreover, these are more consistent and precise than clinical diagnosis by a physician.[1] The American College of Rheumatology (ACR) criteria (1980) has been presented in Table 4.6.[18]

The ACR criteria are limited by its insensitivity to diagnose lSSc, as it was based upon the data drawn from the patients with established disease.

Table 4.6 ACR classification criteria for diagnosis of systemic sclerosis

Major criteria	Minor criteria
Scleroderma proximal to metacarpo-phalangeal joints	• Sclerodactyly • Digital pitted scar or pulp atrophy • Bibasilar pulmonary fibrosis

Source: Masi, A. et al., Arthritis. Rheum., 37, 454–462, 1994.

Note: Presence of major criteria or two of the three minor criteria indicates diagnosis of SSc.

Hence, a further set of classification criteria to include early (LeRoy & Medsger, 2001)[19] and very early cases of SSc (EUSTAR, 2009)[20] had been developed (Table 4.7).

The low sensitivity of the ACR criteria and recent advancements in the knowledge about SSc have led to the development of the current classification criteria.[1] It is a scoring system based upon clinical and immunological features (American College of Rheumatology/European League Against Rheumatism criteria; ACR/EULAR, 2013) (Table 4.8).[1] This classification criterion has a higher sensitivity in diagnosing early and limited form of the disease. The detailed descriptions of the items or sub-items of the ACR/EULAR classification criteria have been defined for better understanding.[1] The ACR/EULAR criteria may also be used by clinicians, researchers, and pharmaceutical industries.[1] The highest possible score in this system is 19, and scores ≥ 9 are considered to give a definite diagnosis of SSc provided other diagnostic possibilities are excluded by adequate measures.[1] Total scores of 9 can be attained by the single sufficient criterion or by combination of others.[1]

Differentiation between subsets of SSc

lSSc and dSSc can be differentiated by typical cutaneous features, systemic involvement, and the auto-antibody pattern (Table 4.9).[2]

Assessment of disease severity

The overall disease severity in these patients can be assessed by a SSc severity scale proposed by Medsger et al. in 1999.[21] The purpose of this tool is to assess the disease activity and the resulted damage to individual organ system. This scale was further modified (2003) and has been presented in Table 4.10.[7] The scale can be used in its entirety, or

Table 4.7 Classification criteria for limited cutaneous SSc

Classification criteria	Major	Minor	
LeRoy & Medsger Criteria for Early Disease	Raynaud's phenomenon	SSc-type nailfold capillary pattern SSc selective auto-antibodies (ACA, Anti-Topoisomerase-1, ARA I/III, anti-fibrillarin, anti-PM-Scl)	Objective documentation of Raynaud's phenomenon and one minor criteria OR Subjective evidence of RP and two minor criteria
EUSTAR criteria for very early disease	Raynaud's phenomenon Auto-antibodies (ANA, ACA, Anti-Topoisomerase-1) Diagnostic nailfold capillary changes	Calcinosis Puffy fingers Digital ulcers Esophageal sphincter dysfunction Telangiectasia Ground-glass appearance of lung fields on HRCT of chest	Presence of three major OR Two major, one minor criterion indicates presence of very early SSc

Source: LeRoy, E., and Medsger, T., J. Rheumatol., 28, 1573–1576, 2001; Matucci-Cerinic, M. et al., Ann. Rheum. Dis., 68, 1377–1380, 2009.

Table 4.8 The American College of Rheumatology/European League Against Rheumatism criteria for the classification of systemic sclerosis[a]

Item	Sub-item(s)	Weight/Score[b]
Skin thickening of the fingers of both hands extending proximal to the metacarpo-phalangeal joints (*sufficient criterion*)	—	9
Skin thickening of the fingers (*only count the higher score*)	Puffy fingers	2
	Sclerodactyly of the fingers (distal to the metacarpo-phalangeal joints but proximal to the interphalangeal joints)	4
Fingertip lesions (*only count the higher score*)	Digital tip ulcers	2
	Fingertip pitting scars	3
Telangiectasia	—	2
Abnormal nailfold capillaries	—	2
Pulmonary arterial hypertension and/or interstitial lung disease (*maximum score is 2*)	Pulmonary arterial hypertension	2
	Interstitial lung disease	2
Raynaud's phenomenon	—	3
SSc-related auto-antibodies (anti-centromere, anti-topoisomerase-I [anti-Scl-70], anti-RNA polymerase-III (*maximum score is 3*)	Anti-centromere Anti-topoisomerase-I Anti-RNA polymerase-III	3

Source: van den Hoogen, F. et al., *Ann. Rheum. Dis.*, 72, 1747–1755, 2013.

[a] These criteria are applicable to any patient considered for inclusion in SSc study. The criteria are not applicable to patients with skin thickening sparing the fingers or to patients who have scleroderma-like disorder that better explains their manifestations (e.g., nephrogenic sclerosing fibrosis, generalized morphea, eosinophilic fasciitis, scleredema diabeticorum, scleromyxedema, erythromyalgia, porphyria, lichen sclerosus, graft-versus-host disease, diabetic cheiroarthropathy).

[b] The total score is determined by adding the maximum weight (score) in each category. Patients with a total score of ≥9 are classified as having definite SSc.

Table 4.9 Characteristics of lSSc and dSSc

Characteristics	lSSc	dSSc
Onset	Slow	Rapid
Progression	Slow progression	Rapid progression
Cutaneous sclerosis	Distal extremities and face mRSS < 14	Extension proximal to elbows and knees, trunk mRSS > 14
Raynaud's phenomenon	Long-term history of Raynaud's phenomenon	Short-term history or concomitant occurrence of Raynaud's phenomenon
Digital ulcers	+	+
Calcinosis	+	
Renal involvement	Low risk for scleroderma-renal crisis	At risk for scleroderma-renal crisis (Anti-RNA polymerase antibody +)
Pulmonary	Isolated/primary pulmonary arterial hypertension	Pulmonary fibrosis/secondary pulmonary hypertension
Gastro-intestinal	Gastro-esophageal reflux disease is universal	
Auto-antibody	Anti-centromere antibody + (50%)	Anti-RNA polymerase antibody + (25%) Anti-topoisomerase antibody + (30%)

Source: Orteu, C.H., and Denton, C.P., Systemic sclerosis, in: Griffiths, C. et al. Eds., *Rook's Textbook of Dermatology*, vol. 2, 9th ed., Wiley Blackwell, Oxford, UK, 56.1–56.23, 2016.

Table 4.10 Revised preliminary SSc severity scale

Organ system	0 (Normal)	1 (Mild)	2 (Moderate)	3 (Severe)	4 (End stage)
1. General	Wt loss < 5%; PCV 37.0%+; Hb 12.3 + Gm/dL	Wt loss 5.0%–9.9%; PCV 33.0%–36.9%; Hb 11.0–12.2 Gm/dL	Wt loss 10.0%–14.9%; PCV 29.0%–32.9%; Hb 9.7–10.9 Gm/dL	Wt loss 15%–19.9%; PCV 25.0%–28.9%; Hb 8.3–9.6 Gm/dL	Wt loss 20+%; PCV <25.0%; Hb <8.3 Gm/dL
2. Peripheral vascular	No Raynaud's; Raynaud's not requiring vasodilators	Raynaud's requiring vasodilators	Digital pitting scars	Digital tip ulcerations	Digital gangrene
3. Skin	TSS 0	TSS 1–14	TSS 15–29	TSS 30–39	TSS 40+
4. Joint/Tendon	FTP 0–0.09 cm	FTP 1.0–1.9 cm	FTP 2.0–3.9 cm	FTP 4.0–4.9 cm	FTP 5.0+ cm
5. Muscle	Normal proximal muscle strength	Proximal weakness, mild	Proximal weakness, moderate	Proximal weakness, severe	Ambulation aids required
6. GI Tract	Normal esophagogram; normal small bowel series	Distal esophageal hypoperistalsis; small bowel series abnormal	Antibiotics required for bacterial overgrowth	Malabsorption syndrome; episodes of pseudoobstruction	Hyperalimentation required
7. Lung	DLCO 80+%; FVC 80+% No fibrosis on radiograph sPAP < 35 mmHg	DLCO 70%–79%; FVC 70%–79%; basilar rales; fibrosis on radiograph; sPAP 35–49 mmHg	DLCO 50%–69%; FVC 50%–69% sPAP 50–64 mmHg	DLCO <50%; FVC < 50% sPAP 65+mmHg	Oxygen required
8. Heart	EKG Normal LVEF 50+%	EKG conduction defect; LVEF 45%–49%	EKG arrhythmia; LVEF 40%–44%	EKG arrhythmia requiring Rx; LVEF 30%–40%	CHF; LVEF < 30%
9. Kidney	No Hx SRC with serum creatinine < 1.3 mg/dL	Hx SRC with serum creatinine < 1.5 mg/dL	Hx SRC with serum creatinine 1.5–2.4 mg/dL	Hx SRC with serum creatinine 2.5–5 mg/dL	Hx SRC with serum creatinine > 5.0 mg/dL or dialysis required

Source: Medsger, T.A. et al., *Clin. Exp. Rheumatol.,* 21, S42–S46, 2003.

Abbreviations: Wt: Weight; PCV: Packed cell volume (hematocrit); Hb: Hemoglobin; TSS: Total skin thickness score; FTP: Fingertip-to-palm distance in flexion; DLCO: Diffusion capacity for carbon monoxide, % predicted; sPAP: estimated pulmonary artery systolic pressure by Doppler echo; EKG: Electrocardiogram; LVEF: left ventricular ejection fraction; Rx:treatment; CHF: congestive heart failure; Hx: history of; SRC: scleroderma renal crisis.

Note: N.B. If two items are included for a severity grade, only one is required for the patient to be scored as having that severity level.

a component of it can be utilized for a given patient to determine particular organ-based severity. Assessment of the disease severity helps in making therapeutic decision and intervention; as early inflammatory stage of SSc is more amenable to therapeutic measures than the late fibrotic phase.

ASSESSMENT OF MORBIDITY

SSc is a progressively debilitating disorder causing physical and social isolation of the patient. It is inevitably associated with significant disease-related morbidity. Adverse events related to prolonged therapy may be additive to this. Many tools have been used to measure the quality of life in these patients. Severity of RP can be assessed by using the Visual Analogue Scale (VAS) or Scleroderma Health Assessment Questionnaire (SHAQ).[7] Scleroderma health associated questionnaire-VAS (SHAQ-VAS) is a scale that can be organ specific, e.g., for gastrointestinal tract (SHAQ-GI-VAS) or lungs.[7] The most commonly used tool for skin involvement is the HAQ-Disability index (HAQ-DI).[7] The HAQ-DI scores correlate with various factors like skin sclerosis, inability to close fists, proximal muscle weakness, and tendon friction rub.[22] SHAQ "global" VAS is also an equally effective tool in this regard.[7] SKindex-29 is a good measure and correlated with patient reported skin symptoms and mRSS.[23]

REFERENCES

1. van den Hoogen F, Khanna D, Fransen J et al. 2013 classification criteria for systemic sclerosis: An American college of rheumatology/European league against rheumatism collaboration initiative. *Ann Rheum Dis* 2013;72:1747–1755.
2. Orteu CH, Denton CP. Systemic sclerosis. In: Griffiths C, Barker J, Bleiker T, Chalmers R, Creamer D, Eds. *Rook's Textbook of Dermatology*, Vol. 2, 9th ed. Oxford, UK: Wiley Blackwell, 2016, pp. 56.1–56.23.
3. Moinzadeh P, Denton CP, Krieg T, Black CM. Scleroderma. In: Goldsmith LA, Katz SI, Gilchrest BA, Paller AS, Leffell DJ, Wolff K, Eds. *Fitzpatrick's Dermatology in General Medicine*, Vol 2, 8th ed. New York: McGraw-Hill Medical, 2012, pp. 1942–1956.
4. Boin F, Wigley FM. Clinical features and treatment of scleroderma. In: Firestein GS, Budd RC, Gabriel SE, McInnes IB, O'Dell JR, Eds. *Kelley's Textbook of Rheumatology*, Vol. 2, 9th ed. Philadelphia, PA: Elsevier Saunders, 2013, pp. 1363–1403.
5. Goodfield M, Dutz J, McCourt C. Lupus erythematosus. In: Griffiths C, Barker J, Bleiker T, Chalmers R, Creamer D, Eds. *Rook's Textbook of Dermatology*, Vol. 2, 9th ed. Oxford, UK: Wiley Blackwell, 2016, pp. 51.1–51.39.
6. Steen VD, Medsger Jr TA. Improvement in skin thickening in systemic sclerosis associated with improved survival. *Arthritis Rheum* 2001;44:2828–2835.
7. Medsger TA, Bombardieri S, Czirjak L, Scorza R, Della Rossa A, Bencivelli W. Assessment of disease severity and prognosis. *Clin Exp Rheumatol* 2003;21:S42–S46.
8. Nikpour M, Stevens WM, Herrick AL, Proudman SM. Epidemiology of systemic sclerosis. *Best Pract Res Clin Rheumatol* 2010;24:857–869.
9. Jaworsky C, Winfield H. Connective tissue diseases. In: Elder DE, Ed. *Lever's Histopathology of the Skin*, 10th ed. Philadelphia, PA: Lippincott Williams & Wilkins, 2009, pp. 279–310.
10. Herrick AL, Clark S. Quantifying digital vascular disease in patients with primary Raynaud's phenomenon and systemic sclerosis. *Ann Rheum Dis* 1998;57:70–78.
11. Naidu S, Baskerville PA, Goss DE, Roberts VC. Raynaud's phenomenon and cold stress testing: A new approach. *Eur J Vas Surg* 1994;8:567–573.
12. Vayssairat M, Evenou P, Baudot N, Priollet P, Gilard M. A new cold test for the diagnosis of Raynaud's phenomenon. *Ann Vas Surg* 1987;1:474–478.
13. Cutolo M, Pizzorni C, Tuccio M et al. Nailfold video-capillaroscopic patterns and serum autoantibodies in systemic sclerosis. *Rheumatology* 2004;43:719–726.
14. Sandqvist G, Eklund M. Hand mobility in scleroderma (HAMIS) test: The reliability of a novel hand function test. *Arthritis Care Res* 2000;13:369–374.
15. Brower LM, Poole JL. Reliability and validity of the Duruoz hand index in persons with systemic sclerosis (scleroderma). *Arthritis Rheum* 2004;51:805–809. Erratum in: *Arthritis Rheum* 2004;53:303.

16. Goh NSL, Desai SR, Veeraraghavan S et al. Interstitial lung disease in systemic sclerosis: A simple staging system. *Am J Respir Crit Care Med* 2008;177:1248–1254.

17. Coghlan JG, Denton CP, Grunig E et al. Evidence-based detection of pulmonary arterial hypertension in systemic sclerosis: The DETECT study. *Ann Rheum Dis* 2014;73:1340–1349.

18. Masi A, Rodnan G, Medsger T. Preliminary criteria for the classification of systemic sclerosis (scleroderma). *Arthritis Rheum* 1994;37:454–462.

19. LeRoy E, Medsger T. Criteria for the classification of early systemic sclerosis. *J Rheumatol* 2001;28:1573–1576.

20. Matucci-Cerinic M, Allanore Y, Czirjak L et al. The challenge of early systemic sclerosis for the EULAR Scleroderma Trial and Research Group (EUSTAR) community. It is time to cut the Gordian knot and develop a prevention of rescue strategy. *Ann Rheum Dis* 2009;68:1377–1380.

21. Medsger TA, JR, Silman AJ, Stehen VD et al. A disease severity scale for systemic sclerosis: Development and testing. *J Rheumatol* 1999;26:2159–2167.

22. Steen VD, Medsger TA Jr. The value of health assessment questionnaire and special patient generated scales to demonstrate change in patients with systemic sclerosis over time. *Arthritis Rheum* 1997;40:1984–1991.

23. Ziemek J, Man A, Hinchcliff M, Varga J, Simms RW, Lafyatis R. The relationship between skin symptoms and the scleroderma modification of the health assessment questionnaire, the modified Rodnan skin score, and skin pathology in patients with systemic sclerosis. *Rheumatology (Oxford)* 2016;55:911–917.

5

Differential diagnoses of systemic sclerosis

KESHAVMURTHY A. ADYA

INTRODUCTION

Systemic sclerosis (SSc) is an autoimmune disorder characterized by multisystem fibrosis associated with vasculopathy and inflammation. The hallmark manifestations of SSc are Raynaud's phenomenon, digital ischemic ulcers, and multiorgan fibrosis. The latter involve the skin and leads to its thickening, termed as "scleroderma." Scleroderma in SSc is bilaterally symmetrical and, in addition to Raynaud's phenomenon, is also associated with antinuclear antibodies (ANA) and specific nailfold capillary changes. When the scleroderma lacks a symmetrical pattern or is not associated with the latter features, other conditions that exhibit skin thickening (scleroderma mimics) must be considered. These account for a myriad group of disorders whose management and prognosis differ from SSc.

DIFFERENTIAL DIAGNOSIS

Sclerosis of the skin dominates the clinical picture of SSc, which may be a feature of many other disorders as well. The other disorders lack the typical systemic and laboratory abnormalities of SSc and are also referred to as sclerodermatous disorders or "pseudoscleroderma." Cutaneous sclerosis in SSc, may be localized (peripheral only), or can be extensive (peripheral and truncal) depending on the type of the disease (limited or diffuse cutaneous types, respectively). Hence, it is important to differentiate other conditions presenting with scleroderma, either localized or diffuse, from SSc. Furthermore, certain sclerodermatous disorders have the propensity to evolve into SSc as well (see below), which makes it prudent for their early recognition and management.

DIFFUSE SCLERODERMATOUS DISORDERS MIMICKING SYSTEMIC SCLEROSIS

Systemic sclerosis mostly needs to be differentiated from generalized (Figure 5.1) or diffuse morphea as both share certain cutaneous features (clinical and histopathological). However, these differ immensely in terms of serology and prognosis. Clinically, as well, some features are characteristic of SSc, which enable differentiation between the two conditions (Table 5.1).[1–3]

The disabling pansclerotic morphea of childhood (Figure 5.2) also bears quite a resemblance with SSc. It is characterized by a progressive and mutilating thickening of the skin, fascia, muscles, and bones. In most of the cases, the changes begin before the age of 14 years. Face, scalp, trunk, and extremities are involved with sparing of digits. Raynaud's phenomenon is absent, but arthralgia and joint contractures are frequent. The involvement of the lungs and esophagus has been described.[4]

Isolated primary SSc should also be differentiated from several overlap syndromes and mixed connective tissue disease, wherein features of other collagen vascular disorders co-exist.

Other diffuse sclerodermatous disorders mimicking SSc have been categorized as in Table 5.2. These disorders may resemble different stages of skin changes of SSc (induration, sclerosis, and atrophic stages). These disorders lack the typical clinical and laboratory abnormalities of systemic sclerosis; absence of Raynaud's phenomenon, typical nailfold capillary changes, and SSc-specific serological abnormalities.

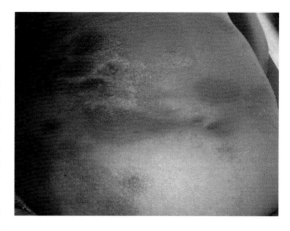

Figure 5.1 Generalized morphoea.

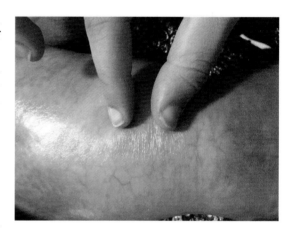

Figure 5.2 Pansclerotic morphoea in a neonate.

Table 5.1 Differentiation between generalized morphea and diffuse systemic sclerosis

Clinical features/serology/prognosis	Generalized morphea	Diffuse systemic sclerosis
Raynaud's phenomenon	Absent	Present
Sites affected by sclerosis	Predominantly trunk	Acral, face and trunk
Sclerodactyly	Absent	Present
Telangiectasia	Absent	Present
Digital pits/scars	Absent	Present
Nailfold capillary changes	Absent	Present
Progressive systemic involvement	Absent[a]	Present
Scl70/Anticentromere antibodies	Absent[b]	Present
Evolution	Usually improves over time	Progressive

[a] Extra-cutaneous manifestations like fever, lymphadenopathy, weakness, arthralgia, and central nervous system involvement may be associated.

[b] Antinuclear antibody positivity and hypergammaglobulinemia may be associated.

Table 5.2 Disorders with diffuse sclerodermatous change in skin

Category	Disorders	Resemblance to stage of SSc
Metabolic and endocrine disorders	Phenylketonuria	Induration
	Diabetes mellitus	Acral sclerosis with limited joint mobility
	Carcinoid syndrome	Induration (initial stage), sclerosis (late stage)
	Muscle glycogenoses[5]	Induration (initial stage), atrophic (late stage)
Deposition disorders	Scleredema	Induration
	Sclerema neonatorum	Induration
	Scleromyxedema	Induration
	Myxedema	Induration
	Primary systemic amyloidosis[6,7]	Sclerosis
Iatrogenic	Graft vs. host disease	Sclerosis
	Drug induced (Table 5.3)	Induration, sclerosis, and joint involvement depending on the drug
Sclerodermatous genodermatoses	Table 5.4	
Occupational	Table 5.5	
Miscellaneous	Eosinophilic fasciitis	Edema followed by induration and sclerosis
	Eosinophilia myalgia syndrome	Edema followed by induration and sclerosis
	Toxic oil syndrome	Edema followed by induration and sclerosis
	Nephrogenic systemic fibrosis	Sclerosis
	Paraneoplastic scleroderma	Sclerosis

Metabolic and endocrine disorders

PHENYLKETONURIA

Phenylketonuria (PKU) is an autosomal recessive disorder due to a deficiency of the enzyme phenylalanine hydroxylase with consequent derangement in phenylalanine and tyrosine metabolism. Principal features of PKU are seizures, mental retardation, microcephaly, and cutaneous changes. Apart from the common pigmentary dilution, eczematous, and sclerodermatous changes in the skin are also seen. Though the scleroderma in most instances is limited, diffuse or even progressive forms with systemic involvement have also been reported. The sclerodermatous changes usually appear in the first two years of life and commonly involve the extremities. Such changes are attributed to the shunting of phenylalanine to a transamination pathway due to the enzyme deficiency; there is overproduction and accumulation of phenylpyruvic acid and its metabolites in the skin. Impaired conversion of tryptophan to 5-hydroxytryptophan leading to increased indole acetic acid and decreased tissue serotonin is also implicated in the development of sclerodermatous skin changes. The changes generally reverse when the patient is on phenylalanine elimination diet.[8–10]

DIABETES MELLITUS

Skin thickening in diabetes mellitus can occur in three forms; generalized asymptomatic skin thickening, (Figure 5.3) thickening of the dorsum of the hands and fingers, and scleredema diabeticorum. Involvement of the hands and fingers

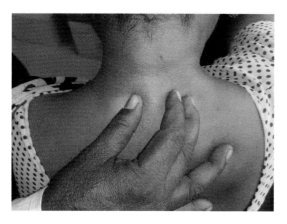

Figure 5.3 Scleredema diabeticorum. (Courtesy of Dr. Chetan Rajput.)

is characteristic and is seen in both forms of the disease. The thickening may range from localized involving only the knuckles, to the diabetic hand syndrome. The former is characterized by either pebbling of the entire dorsal surface of the fingers and the periungual region or may be limited to the knuckles (Huntley's papules). The diabetic hand syndrome is characterized by limited mobility of the finger joints together with a thickened and waxy appearance of the skin. Involvement of the metacarpophalangeal and proximal interphalangeal joints is the initial manifestation characterized by a reduced extension of the palm (initially active and later passive). Skin thickening follows the joint manifestations, which are progressive with age. These changes are often associated with an early onset and long duration of diabetes and are attributable to the nonenzymatic glycosylation of the collagen that accumulates and produces microvascular alterations with consequent low-grade tissue ischemia and fibrosis.[11,12]

CARCINOID SYNDROME

Sclerodermatous lesions in carcinoid syndrome are uncommon but well recognized. They usually indicate advanced disease with poor prognosis. Frequently, the mid-gut carcinoids are associated with scleroderma and most of them would have metastasized to the liver at the time of presentation. Excessive serotonin and other vasoactive amines secreted by the tumor are implicated in the development of fibrosis, which may also affect the cardiac and pulmonary valves. Substance P and neurokinin A are also thought to be important mediators of sclerosis, as these are exclusively secreted by the midgut carcinoids and are capable of inducing dermal fibroblast proliferation. The scleroderma almost always involves the lower extremities and improvement with octreotide, cyproheptadine, and prednisolone are reported, although progressive forms have also been documented.[13–16]

Deposition disorders

SCLEREDEMA

Scleredema is a disorder characterized by symmetrically indurated skin due to excessive dermal mucin deposition. Although termed as *scleredema adultorum* (of Buschke) and frequently affecting middle-aged obese adults, children can be affected as well. Etiologically, scleredema can be grouped into diabetes-associated (commonly with uncontrolled type II diabetes mellitus), post-infectious (streptococcal upper respiratory tract infection, influenza, mumps, measles, varicella, cytomegalovirus, diphtheria, encephalitis, and dental abscesses), and with paraproteinemias. Exact pathogenesis of scleredema is unclear. Nonenzymatic glycosylation of collagen and stimulation of fibroblast proliferation by chronic hyperinsulinemia are implicated in diabetic scleredema. The induration is non-pitting and predominantly involves the posterior neck and upper back and may extend on to the face and proximal extremities. The affected area appears erythematous with a *peau d' orange* appearance (mattress sign) and has a woody hard consistency. Scleredema associated with diabetes (scleredema diutinum) and paraproteinemia are usually progressive and unresponsive to treatment. The postinfectious form carries a good prognosis and usually resolves in a few months to couple of years.[17,18]

SCLEREMA NEONATORUM

Although sclerema neonatorum (Figure 5.4) may be a different diagnosis of scleroderma in the pediatric age group, the clinical characteristics are quite distinct to pose any diagnostic difficulty.[19]

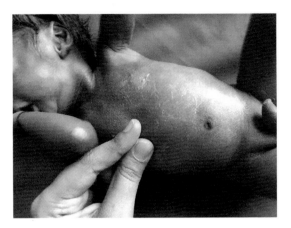

Figure 5.4 Sclerema neonatorum.

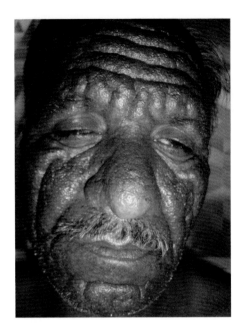

Figure 5.5 Scleromyxedema.

It is a disorder of preterm neonates with an underlying severe illness carrying a poor prognosis. It is characterized by rapidly progressive non-pitting skin hardening due to solidification of saturated fatty acids, which have a low threshold for hypothermia. The hardening initially begins over the buttocks and thighs and spreads to the entire body sparing the palms and soles. Reduced chest expansion and flexion deformities of joints may be present as well. Neonatal sepsis is the most common underlying cause, although cardiovascular disease, pulmonary haemorrhage, central nervous system abnormalities, hypothermia, metabolic acidosis, and glucose or electrolyte imbalances have also been implicated. Prognosis depends on the underlying cause but is poor in most of the cases despite aggressive treatment.

SCLEROMYXEDEMA

Scleromyxedema (Figure 5.5) is a primary cutaneous mucinosis characterized by diffuse or localized dermal mucin infiltration leading to a thickening and a smooth waxy appearance of the skin. The infiltration is often accompanied by smooth waxy, pruritic, closely-set papules. Most of the cases are associated with monoclonal gammopathy. The typical sites involved are the mid-upper back and forehead with deep glabellar furrows. Involvement of the face, forearms, and hands gives a smooth ironed-out appearance, as in SSc. However, such an appearance in SSc is

due to sclerosis rather than infiltration. Further, reduced mouth opening and sclerodactyly due to infiltration also simulates SSc.[17] Severe esophageal dysmotility due to mucin infiltration of the esophageal walls leading to significant dysphagia has also been reported with scleredema.[20]

MYXEDEMA

In severe cases of hypothyroidism, there is excessive accumulation of mucopolysaccharides in the dermis leading to non-pitting induration of the skin, especially involving the face (Figure 5.6), hands, and pretibial areas. Periorbital puffiness, macroglossia, a loss of the lateral one-third of the eyebrows, and generalized xerosis are associated and help in clinical differentiation.[21]

Iatrogenic

GRAFT VERSUS HOST DISEASE

Sclerodermatous lesions can occur in 5%–15% of chronic graft versus host disease (cGVHD) and can either be localized and scattered, or generalized with joint contractures, and esophageal

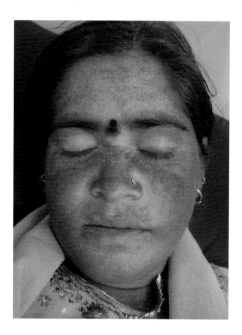

Figure 5.6 Hypothyroidism.

dysmotility simulating dSSc. Nailfold changes similar to SSc can also be found in about 50% of the cases. Sclerodermatous cGVHD is attributed to end-organ fibrosis, and the sclerosis may even involve the subcutaneous fat and underlying fascia unlike the predominantly dermal sclerosis in SSc. The scleroderma is often accompanied by disabling chronic painful ulcers. Sclerodermatous cGVHD is relatively rare but a severe form of the disorder; it is often unresponsive to treatment and associated with poor prognosis.[22–24]

DRUG INDUCED SCLERODERMA

Many drugs have been implicated in the causation of scleroderma-like syndromes. Both localized and diffuse scleroderma-like skin changes can be induced by drugs and drug induced SSc-like syndrome has been described as well. In general, drug induced scleroderma can be distinguished from primary scleroderma/SSc by the following[25]:

- Type of skin lesions (acrosclerosis, localized or diffuse morpheaform lesions, fibrotic nodules, joint contractures),
- Presence of organ damage (renal, hepatic, nervous system, muscles),
- Absent SSc specific autoantibodies, and,
- Reversal of the changes on discontinuation of the drugs.

Among the various drugs, bleomycin-induced scleroderma is frequently encountered. Bleomycin stimulates collagen synthesis in cultured normal skin fibroblasts. The sclerotic changes also involve the lungs causing pulmonary fibrosis and are dependent on cumulative doses administered. Cutaneous sclerosis frequently affects the hands, forearms, arms, thighs, legs, and feet. Raynaud's phenomenon and antinuclear antibody positivity have also been described. Similar changes are seen with cisplatin.[25,26]

Taxane (docetaxel, palcitaxel) induced scleroderma is attributed to *versican*, a proteoglycan that influences the proliferation and migration of fibroblasts as well as synthesis of extracellular matrix, which has been found intensely deposited in the skin after docetaxel administration. Edematous lesions, either as discrete plaques or diffuse lower limb edema, are the characteristic of docetaxel-induced scleroderma that later harden. Joint involvement may also occur.[25,27]

Localized morpheaform lesions following vitamin K injections have been described (Texier's disease). The initial lesions begin as erythematous plaques that progress to pruritic dusky red lesions and eventually become sclerodermatous with typical ivory white central sclerosis and a lilac margin. Lesions developing in the lumbosacral region circumferentially have been described as "cowboy's holster" in appearance.[28]

Release of silica into the surrounding skin following local silicone gel injections for breast augmentation has been associated with a development of either localized morpheform lesions, or a more systemic disease resembling SSc (human adjuvant disease).[29] Table 5.3 enlists other drugs causing scleroderma-like syndromes.[25–30]

Sclerodermatous genodermatoses

These groups of inherited disorders are characterized by unique phenotypic attributes with the cutaneous features resembling different clinical manifestations of SSc. As with any other pseudosclerodermatous condition, absence of Raynaud's phenomenon, nailfold capillary changes, and serological abnormalities help in differentiation. Table 5.4 briefly outlines the sclerodermatous manifestations and other clinical features of such disorders.[31–40]

Table 5.3 Drugs causing diffuse scleroderma-like appearance

Category	Drugs
Chemotherapeutic drugs	Bleomycin
	Cisplatin
	Docetaxel
	Palcitaxel
Analgesics	Morphine
	Penatazocine
	Bromocriptine
	Ergot
	Methysergide
	Ketobemidone
Appetite suppressants	Diethylpropion hydrochloride
	Mazindol
	Amphetamine
	Dexamphetamine
	Phenmetrazine
	Methaqualone
Central nervous system drugs	Carbidopa
	L-5-hydroxy-tryptophan
	Ethosuximide
Others	L-tryptophan
	Beta blockers (bisoprolol)
	ACE inhibitors (Fosinopril)
	D-Penicillamine
	Interferon α
	Interleukin 2
	Anti-TNF agents
	Balicatib
	Cocaine
	Local injections of vitamin K, silicone, paraffin, vitamin B12 and progestin

Abbreviations: ACE: Angiotensin converting enzyme, TNF: Tumor necrosis factor.

Occupational sclerodermatous disorders

Occupational exposures of certain agents produce clinical manifestations that resemble localized or diffuse morphea and/or systemic sclerosis (Table 5.5). Interestingly, certain manifestations of SSc like Raynaud's phenomenon, facial telangiectasia, and nailfold capillary changes may also be associated with some of these disorders though the characteristic serological abnormalities are usually absent, and the manifestations may reverse on discontinuation of the exposure.[29]

Other diffuse sclerodermatous disorders mimicking systemic sclerosis

EOSINOPHILIC FASCIITIS

Eosinophilic fasciitis is a disorder of unclear etiopathogenesis characterized by acute or subacute onset erythema and edema of the extremities, with or without involvement of the trunk. The acral areas are typically spared. The edematous stage is succeeded by induration and fibrosis mimicking scleroderma.

Trauma, drugs, and infective agents (*Borrelia* species) have been implicated, and association with hematologic disorders has also been described. The fibrosis primarily affects the fascia rather than dermis, and there is a presence of peripheral eosinophilia, hypergammaglobulinemia, and raised erythrocyte sedimentation rate. Principal features differentiating eosinophilic fasciitis from SSc are the absence of Raynaud's phenomenon, systemic involvement, and nailfold capillary changes. Prognostically, eosinophilic fasciitis is self-limiting unless associated with hematologic disorders.[41]

EOSINOPHILIA MYALGIA SYNDROME

Eosinophilia myalgia syndrome is related to consumption of L-tryptophan and is characterized by acute or subacute onset of myalgia, arthralgia, edema of the extremities, fever, respiratory symptoms, pulmonary hypertension, arrhythmias, and polyneuropathy. A multitude of cutaneous manifestations may be present; morbilliform exanthem, urticaria, livedo reticularis, and papular mucinosis. Extensive sclerodermatous changes similar to eosinophilic fasciitis are also seen. Peripheral blood eosinophilia is present. The clinical manifestations are due to the impurities in L-tryptophan. A strikingly similar syndrome following consumption of contaminated rapeseed oil was described in Spain in 1981 (the toxic oil syndrome).[42,43]

Table 5.4 Scleroderma-like genodermatoses

Syndrome	Inheritance and genetic defect	Sclerodermatous manifestations	Other predominant manifestations
Premature Aging Syndromes			
Werner's syndrome (Adult progeria)	AR, mutation in *WRN* gene that regulates DNA replication and repair	Sclerosis and atrophy of the distal extremities, especially legs and feet, often accompanied by deformities and ulceration	Premature aging (beginning after puberty), short stature, bird-like facies, thin distal extremities, predisposition to diabetes and hypogonadism, premature death due to atherosclerotic complications
Progeria (Hutchison-Gilford syndrome)	Sporadic autosomal dominant mutation in *LMNA* gene encoding lamin A, an important component of nuclear membrane	Sclerodermatous skin over the limbs and phalanges histologically showing increased dermal collagen	Short stature, disproportionately large head with prominent scalp veins and alopecia. Beaked nose with loss of facial fat and wrinkled skin giving a plucked bird appearance. Profound growth retardation, skeletal deformities, and pronounced features of premature aging beginning at 1–2 years of life are other important features.
Neonatal progeroid syndrome (Wiedemann-Rautenstrauch syndrome)	?AR	Diffuse sclerodermoid changes with contractures of lower extremities	Premature aged appearance at birth with severe growth retardation. Distinctive craniofacial features – triangular face, large skull with prominent veins and wide anterior fontanelle, small face, natal teeth, low-set posteriorly rotated ears, ectropion, and hypotrichosis
Acrogeria (Gottron syndrome)	?AR	Thin, taut, and parchment-like acral skin.	Other features may include abnormally small hands and feet, prominent veins on the chest, micrognathia, and short stature.
Poikilodermatous Syndromes			
Hereditary sclerosing poikiloderma (of Weary)	AD trait with incomplete penetrance	Sclerosis of palms and soles, linear hyperkeratotic and sclerotic bands in the axillae, and antecubital and popliteal fossae	Other features include generalized poikiloderma with accentuation in flexures, finger clubbing, aortic valve calcification, and tissue calcinosis

(Continued)

Table 5.4 (Continued) Scleroderma-like genodermatoses

Syndrome	Inheritance and genetic defect	Sclerodermatous manifestations	Other predominant manifestations
Hereditary mandibuloacral dysplasia	AR, mutations in the lamin A/C (LMNA) and zinc metalloproteinase (ZMPSTE24) genes in types A and B, respectively	Distinct scleroderma-like changes with finger contractures and sclerosing poikiloderma	Progeroid features with dysplastic mandible, clavicle, bulbous digits, and lipodystrophy with accompanying metabolic syndrome
Other Genodermatoses			
Congenital fascial dystrophy (stiff skin syndrome) (Figure 5.7)	AR, mutation in FBN1 gene that regulates TGF-β2 production	Stony hard sclerosis of the skin prominently over the buttocks and thighs with "cobble-stoning;" diffuse progressive sclerosis in the "Parana" type.	Restricted joint mobility and lung movements, variable hypertrichosis, typical "tip-toe" posture, and exaggerated lumbar lordosis
GEMMS syndrome	AD	Thickened skin due to excessive production of normal collagen possibly due to TGF-β1 over-activity	Glaucoma, ectopia lentis, microspherophakia, joint stiffness, and short stature
Scleroatrophy of Huriez	AD	Scleroatrophy of the hands with hypoplastic nails	Palmoplantar keratoderma with absent dermatoglyphics, increased risk of squamous cell carcinoma
Familial sclerodermatous finger deformity		Familial scleroderma-like deformity of the distal phalanges with vascular symptoms suggestive of Raynaud's phenomenon, and scleroderma-like changes of the fingers with psoriasiform dermatitis with nail plate shortening and restricted joint mobility have been described	
Moore-Federman syndrome and acromicric dysplasia	AD	Skin thickening (of the extremities)	Dwarfism, hypermetropia, asthma, and stiffness of hand joints in Moore-Federman syndrome. Additionally, characteristic facies (narrow palpebral fissures with short stubby nose and anteverted nostrils) in acromicric dysplasia

Abbreviations: AR: Autosomal recessive, AD: Autosomal dominant, TGF: Transforming, growth factor, GEMSS: Glaucoma, ectopia lentis, microspherophakia, joint stiffness, and short stature.

Table 5.5 Occupational scleroderma-like disorders

Occupation	Exposure agents	Sclerodermatous features	Other features
Reactor cleaners, PVC workers	Polyvinyl chloride (vinyl chloride disease)	Cold, stiff, numb, fingers, hands, and feet with burning pain and discoloration on cold exposure. Facial telangiectases and nail fold capillary changes similar to those seen in SSc can occur.	Lethargy, loss of libido, impotence, dyspnoea, and hepatosplenomegaly. X-ray: Erosion of terminal phalanges, metatarsals, pelvic bones, clavicles, and bones of the arms and legs.
Dry cleaners and solvent handlers	Benzene, toluenes, toluidines, xylenes, xylidenes, aniline compounds, perchloroethylene, trichloroethylene, ethyl acetate, naphthalene, ethanolamine, isopropyl alcohol, trimethylbenzene, terpene derivatives, and phenylenediamine	Similar to vinyl chloride disease	Systemic features like restrictive lung defect, peripheral neuropathy, esophageal dysfunction, hypertension, and paraproteinaemia
Farmers and pesticide handlers	Chlordane, heptochlor, DDT, malathion, parathion, sodium dinitro-orthocresolate, and 7-chlorocyclohexane	Sclerodermatous changes with Raynaud's phenomenon	
Miners	Silica	SSc-like features indistinguishable from idiopathic type	Accompanied or preceded by silicosis
Transformer workers	Epoxy resins	Scleroderma-like skin changes and erythema, with fatigue, loss of weight, myalgia and arthralgia	

Abbreviations: PVC: Polyvinyl chloride, SSc: Systemic sclerosis, DDT: Dichlorodiphenyltrichloroethane.

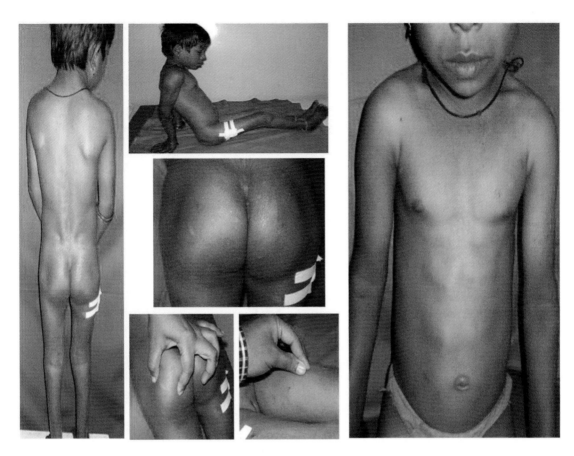

Figure 5.7 Stiff skin syndrome in a child.

NEPHROGENIC SYSTEMIC FIBROSIS

Nephrogenic systemic fibrosis (nephrogenic fibrosing dermopathy) is characterized by induration and sclerosis predominantly involving the extremities (Figure 5.8a and b), either in a localized or diffuse manner, occurring in patients with renal compromise who are subjected to gadolinium exposure during imaging studies. The skin in the affected area has a shiny look and a woody hard consistency, and is usually associated with hyperpigmentation, surface alterations like *peau d' orange* appearance, and fibrotic subcutaneous nodules. Localized plaques characteristically exhibit amoeboid projections from the margins. Histologically, features reminiscent of scleredema are seen.[44]

Malignancy-associated (paraneoplastic) scleroderma

Increased risk of hematological and solid organ malignancies in patients with SSc, compared to the general population, is well established.[45] Sclerodermatous changes as paraneoplastic manifestations are also described with various malignancies. Such changes are frequently described with carcinoid syndrome (see above), malignancies of the breast, uterus, lungs, stomach, nasopharynx, and melanoma. Sclerodermatous lesions are also associated with plasma cell dyscrasias, including multiple myeloma, Waldenström macroglobulinemia, and the Crow-Fukase syndrome.[46–48]

The sclerodermatous manifestations can either be diffuse or localized morpheaform, or SSc-like with Raynaud's phenomenon and are attributed to the release of mediators by tumor cells identical to those seen in the sera of patients with idiopathic SSc. Increased levels of circulating anti-topoisomerase I antibodies are frequently associated with paraneoplastic scleroderma.

In general, the occurrence of scleroderma after 50 years of age associated with sclerodactyly, progressive cutaneous sclerosis, and rapid

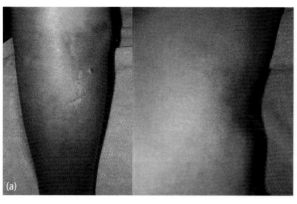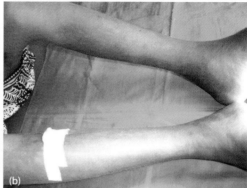

Figure 5.8 **(a, b)** Nephrogenic systemic fibrosis.

onset Raynaud's phenomenon are indicative of the paraneoplastic form. Such features in the absence of Raynaud's phenomenon with a normal capillaroscopy pattern are also indicative of paraneoplastic rather than idiopathic scleroderma.[49] In contrast to other paraneoplastic phenomena, treatment of underlying malignancy does not lead to regression of the sclerodermatous changes.[50]

LOCALIZED SCLERODERMATOUS DISORDERS MIMICKING SYSTEMIC SCLEROSIS

Localized asymmetrical thickening of the skin may also be seen in SSc when other disorders with such manifestations may have to be differentiated. All variants of morphea (circumscribed, guttate, linear, subcutaneous, and frontoparietal) have to be primarily differentiated. Circumscribed morphea occur as single or multiple ivory-white sclerotic plaques with a lilac margin in active stage and as hyperpigmented atrophic plaques in regressing stage. Linear morphea is common in childhood and frequently involve an extremity.[29]

About 10% cases of porphyria cutanea tarda show sclerodermatous changes; either localized morpheaform (involving both the photo-exposed and covered areas) or generalized with sclerodactyly and joint contracture.[25]

Localized morphea has also been described with hepatitis C infection.[51–54] Scleroderma associated with GVHD, drugs, occupational chemical exposure, nephrogenic systemic fibrosis,

and carcinoid syndrome may also be localized as described above.

CONCLUSION

Myriads of sclerodermatous disorders mimic primary SSc. It is prudent to have an in-depth knowledge of such conditions to enable appropriate evaluation, ascertaining the prognosis, and management of such disorders.

REFERENCES

1. Zulian F. Systemic manifestations in localized scleroderma. *Curr Rheumatol Rep* 2004;6:417–424.
2. Chung L, Lin J, Furst DE, Fiorentino D. Systemic and localized scleroderma. *Clin Dermatol* 2006;24:374–392.
3. Leitenberger JJ, Cayce RL, Haley RW, Adams-Huet B, Bergstresser PR, Jacobe HT. Distinct autoimmune syndromes in morphea: A review of 245 adult and pediatric cases. *Arch Dermatol* 2009;145:545–550.
4. Diaz-Perez JL, Connolly SM, Winkelmann RK. Disabling pansclerotic morphoea of children. *Arch Dermatol* 1980;116:169–173.
5. Jablonska S, Stachow A. Pseudoscleroderma concomitant with a muscular glycogenosis of unknown enzymatic defect. *Acta Derm Venereol (Stockh)* 1972;52:379–385.

6. Sun L, Zhang L, Hu W, Li TF, Liu S. One case of primary AL amyloidosis repeatedly misdiagnosed as scleroderma. *Medicine* 2017;96:50(e8771).

7. Reyes CM, Rudinskaya A, Kloss R, Girardi M, Lazova R. Scleroderma-like illness as a presenting feature of multiple myeloma and amyloidosis. *J Clin Rheumatol* 2008;14:161–165.

8. Al-Mayouf SM, Al-Owain MA. Progressive sclerodermatous skin changes in a child with phenylketonuria. *Pediatr Dermatol* 2006;23:136–138.

9. Haktan M, Aydin A, Bahat H, Tuysuz B, Yazici H, Altay S. Progressive systemic scleroderma in an infant with partial phenylketonuria. *J Inherit Metab Dis* 1989;12:486–487.

10. Nova MP, Kaufman M, Halperin A. Scleroderma-like skin indurations in a child with phenylketonuria: A clinicopathologic correlation and review of the literature. *J Am Acad Dermatol* 1992;26:329–333.

11. Van Hattem S, Bootsma AH, Thio HB. Skin manifestations of diabetes. *Cleve Clin J Med* 2008;75:772, 774, 776–777.

12. Upreti V, Vasdev V, Dhull P, Patnaik SK. Prayer sign in diabetes mellitus. *Indian J Endocr Metab* 2013;17:769–770.

13. Bell HK, Poston GJ, Vora J, Wilson NJ. Cutaneous manifestations of the malignant carcinoid syndrome. *Br J Dermatol* 2005;152:71–75.

14. Durward G, Blackford S, Roberts D, Jones MK. Cutaneous scleroderma in association with carcinoid syndrome. *Postgrad Med J* 1995;71:299–300.

15. Mota JM, Sousa LG, Riechelmann RP. Complications from carcinoid syndrome: Review of the current evidence. *Ecancermedicalscience* 2016;10:662.

16. Mattingly PC, Mowat AG. Rapidly progressive scleroderma associated with carcinoma of the oesophagus. *Ann Rheum Dis* 1979;38:177–178.

17. Tyndall A, Fistarol S. The differential diagnosis of systemic sclerosis. *Curr Opin Rheumatol* 2013;25:692–699.

18. Rongioletti F. Cutaneous mucinosis. In: Griffiths CEM, Barker J, Bleiker T, Chalmers R, Creamer D, Eds. *Rook's Textbook of Dermatology*, 9th ed. Oxford, UK: Wiley-Blackwell, 2016, pp. 59.1–59.18.

19. Adya KA, Inamadar AC. Skin of the newborn: Physiological and pathological changes. In: Gupta P, Menon PSN, Ramji S, Lodha R, Eds. *PG Textbook of Pediatrics*, 1st ed. New Delhi, India: Jaypee Brothers Medical Publishers, 2015, pp. 2646–2653.

20. Chatterjee S, Hedman BJ, Kirby DF. An unusual cause of dysphagia. *J Clin Rheumatol* 2018;24:444–448.

21. Lause M, Kamboj A, Fernandez Faith E. Dermatologic manifestations of endocrine disorders. *Transl Pediatr* 2017;6:300–312.

22. Scheinfeld NS. Dermatologic manifestations of graft versus host disease. Available at https://emedicine.medscape.com/article/1050580-overview#a3. Accessed January 10, 2018.

23. Kitko CL, White ES, Baird K. Fibrotic and sclerotic manifestations of chronic graft-versus-host disease. *Biol Blood Marrow Transplant* 2012;18(1 Suppl):S46–S52.

24. Jedlickova Z, Burlakova I, Bug G, Baurmann H, Schwerdtfeger R, Schleuning M. Therapy of sclerodermatous chronic graft-versus-host disease with mammalian target of rapamycin inhibitors. *Biol Blood Marrow Transplant* 2011;17:657–663.

25. Haustein UF, Haupt B. Drug-induced scleroderma and sclerodermiform conditions. *Clin Dermatol* 1998;16:353–366.

26. Finch WR, Rodnan GP, Buckingham RB, Prince RK, Winkelstein A. Bleomycin-induced scleroderma. *J Rheumatol* 1980;7:651–659.

27. Okada K, Endo Y, Miyachi Y, Koike Y, Kuwatsuka Y, Utani A. Glycosaminoglycan and versican deposits in taxane-induced sclerosis. *Br J Dermatol* 2015;173:1054–1058.

28. Pang BK, Munro V, Kossard S. Pseudoscleroderma secondary to phytomenadione (vitamin K1) injections: Texier's disease. *Australas J Dermatol* 1996;37:44–47.

29. Goodfield MJD, Jones SK, Veale DJ. The "Connective tissue diseases." In: Burns T, Breathnach S, Cox N, Griffiths C, Eds. *Rook's Textbook of Dermatology*, 8th ed. Oxford, UK: Wiley-Blackwell, 2010, pp. 51.1–51.138.

30. Mauduit G, Cambazard F, Faure M, Thivolet J. Pseudoscleroderma and sclerodermiform states. *Ann Med Interne (Paris)* 1984;135:615–623.
31. Haustein UF. Scleroderma and pseudo-scleroderma: uncommon presentations. *Clin Dermatol* 2005;23:480–490.
32. Werner syndrome. Available at https://ghr.nlm.nih.gov/condition/werner-syndrome. Accessed on January 20, 2018.
33. Jablonska S, Blaszczyk M. Scleroderma-like disorders. *Semin Cutan Med Surg* 1998;17:65–76.
34. Neonatal progeroid syndrome. Available at https://rarediseases.info.nih.gov/diseases/330/neonatal-progeroid-syndrome. Accessed on January 21, 2018.
35. Poikiloderma, hereditary sclerosing. Available at https://omim.org/entry/173700. Accessed on January 21, 2018.
36. Mandibuloacral dysplasia. Available at https://rarediseases.org/rare-diseases/mandibuloacral-dysplasia/. Accessed on January 21, 2018.
37. Amorim AGF, Aide MK, Duraes SMB, Rochael MC. Stiff skin syndrome: A case report. *An Bras Dermatol* 2011;86(S1):S178–S181.
38. Cat I, Magdalena NI, Marinoni LP et al. Parana hard-skin syndrome: Study of seven families. *Lancet* 1974;303:215–216.
39. Kunz M, Paulus W, Sollberg S et al. Sclerosis of the skin in the GEMSS syndrome. An overproduction of normal collagen. *Arch Dermatol* 1995;131:1170–1174.
40. Winter RM, Patton MA, Challener J, Mueller RF, Baraitser M. Moore-Federman syndrome and acromicric dysplasia: Are they the same entity? *J Med Genet* 1989;26:320–325.
41. Henning PM, Mount GR, Kortan ND, Nasef S, Lohr KM. Eosinophilic fasciitis. Available at https://emedicine.medscape.com/article/329515-overview. Accessed on January 29, 2018.
42. Monaco WE, Mathew SD. Eosiniphilia-myalgia syndrome. Available at https://emedicine.medscape.com/article/329614-overview. Accessed on January 29, 2018.
43. Iglesias JL, De Moragas JM. The cutaneous lesions of the Spanish toxic oil syndrome. *J Am Acad Dermatol* 1983;9:159–160.
44. Scheinfeld NS, Cowper S. Nephrogenic systemic fibrosis. Available at https://emedicine.medscape.com/article/1097889-overview. Accessed on January 29, 2018.
45. Zeineddine N, Khoury LE, Mosak J. Systemic sclerosis and malignancy: A review of current data. *J Clin Med Res* 2016;8:625–632.
46. Jedlickova H, Durčanská V, Vašků V. Paraneoplastic scleroderma: Are there any clues? *Acta Dermatovenerol Croat* 2016;24:78–80.
47. Ciołkiewicz M, Domysławska I, Ciołkiewicz A, Klimiuk PA, Kuryliszyn-Moskal A. Coexistence of systemic sclerosis, scleroderma-like syndromes and neoplastic diseases. *Pol Arch Med Wewn* 2008;118:119–126.
48. Magro CM, Iwenofu H, Nuovo GJ. Paraneoplastic scleroderma-like tissue reactions in the setting of an underlying plasma cell dyscrasia: A report of 10 cases. *Am J Dermatopathol* 2013;35:561–568.
49. Racanelli V, Prete M, Minoia C, Favoino E, Perosa F. Rheumatic disorders as paraneoplastic syndromes. *Autoimmun Rev* 2008;7:352–358.
50. Launay D, Le Berre R, Hatron PY et al. Association between systemic sclerosis and breast cancer: Eight new cases and review of the literature. *Clin Rheumatol* 2004;23:516–522.
51. de Oliveira FL, de Barros Silveira LK, Rambaldi ML, Barbosa FC. Localized scleroderma associated with chronic hepatitis C. *Case Rep Dermatol Med* 2012;2012:743896.
52. Jackson JM, Callen JP. Scarring alopecia and sclerodermatous changes of the scalp in a patient with hepatitis C infection. *J Am Acad Dermatol* 1998;39:824–826.
53. Mihas AA, Abou-Assi SG, Heuman DM. Cutae morphea associated with chronic hepatitis C. *J Hepatol* 2003;39:458–459.
54. Telakis E, Nikolaou A. Localized scleroderma (morphea) in a patient with chronic hepatitis C. *Eur J Gastroenterol Hepatol* 2009;21:486.

6

Management of scleroderma

KESHAVMURTHY A. ADYA

INTRODUCTION

The management of scleroderma is essentially aimed at the disease complications as and when these arise. The main components of the disease, the fibrosis and vasculopathy result in specific organ damage. The natural history of the disease is progressive, with acute events in the form of renal and pulmonary complications. The existing therapeutic options are more of symptom-alleviating and do not cause reversal of the disease process. Hence, life-style modifications and other symptom-oriented general interventions play a large role in the management of this disorder. This calls for patient participation and cooperation from family members in a great way in parallel with the therapeutic interventions.

Treatment measures significantly improve the quality of life in these patients and reduce the morbidity. Therapy of localized cutaneous disease and organ-specific managements in diffuse disease have been discussed below.

MANAGEMENT OF MORPHEA

In localized or diffuse morphea, the main aims of treatment are:

- To prevent development of sclerosis in the early inflammatory stage
- To prevent the progression of sclerosis and atrophy in established cases

Treatment of morphea is essentially guided by the disease type, extent, and activity. Circumscribed or localized morphea with limited cutaneous involvement can be managed with topical and/or intralesional therapy; whereas, linear and diffuse morphea require a relatively aggressive systemic therapeutic approach as these may potentially lead to permanent disfigurement. In any case though, the endeavor should be to initiate treatment early in the inflammatory stage of the disease and prevent development of sclerosis rather than attempting to reverse the latter.

Treatment of localized and limited morphea

In the early inflammatory stage, topical or intralesional corticosteroids are recommended. Alternatively, topical tacrolimus, calcipotriol, or imiquimod have also been used. Cases not responding to these initial measures are treated with combination therapies like calcipotriol with betamethasone, imiquimod. Low-dose ultraviolet-A (UVA) phototherapy alone or in combination with calcipotriol can be used. Such therapy decreases the inflammation and halts the disease progression. Sequels like pigmentory changes are inevitable. In burnt out cases, management of atrophy can be achieved with plastic and cosmetic surgical techniques.[1–5]

Treatment of diffuse and linear morphea

Diffuse and linear morphea require aggressive systemic treatment as joint contractures and associated morbidity is significant, especially with the latter. The initial recommended treatment in active disease include systemic corticosteroids (prednisolone 0.5–1 mg/kg/d or pulsed methyl prednisolone 30 mg/kg 3 days in a week) or methotrexate (maximum dose of 25 mg/week). Corticosteroids and methotrexate can be used as monotherapy or in combination. Mycophenolate mofetil is recommended as an option in patients intolerant or unresponsive to methotrexate.[6,7] Phototherapy with UVA (with or without psoralens) and narrowband ultraviolet B (NB-UVB) are the other safer and useful therapeutic options. Recently, biologicals have been used in these patients with significant improvement; these include, the tumor necrosis factor α (TNF α) antibody and tyrosine kinase inhibitors.[8,9] In patients with established joint contractures and deformities, physiotherapy and plastic reconstructive surgeries are recommended.[1]

MANAGEMENT OF SYSTEMIC SCLEROSIS

Management of systemic sclerosis (SSc) has three aims:

- Treatment of clinical manifestations due to involvement of various systems

- General and specific measures for management of cutaneous manifestations/complications
- Specific systemic immunosuppressive therapy to prevent progression of the disease

Management of SSc may prevent progressive systemic fibrosis and microvascular damage; at the same time, judicious management of the complications arising due to the involvement of various organs including skin ensures a better quality of life.

Management of cutaneous vasculopathic manifestations

RAYNAUD'S PHENOMENON

Repeated episodes of painful Raynaud's phenomenon (RP) are debilitating for the patients with SSc, affecting their quality of life significantly. Life style modification and avoidance of known precipitating factors play an important role in prevention of SSc-associated RP. These include keeping the extremities warm using woollen gloves and socks regularly; avoidance of handling cold water; and, staying away from high altitudes and exposure to cold climates as far as practicable. Electric, re-warming devices for keeping the extremities warm can be used when available. In addition, factors that induce vasospasm like emotional stress, smoking, and cold beverages must also be avoided. Drugs that may induce vasospasm, like sympathomimetics, serotonin agonists used for migraine, and non-selective beta blockers (propranolol) must be avoided.[10]

Calcium channel blockers (nifedipine, nicardipine, amlodipine, nislodipine) are recommended as a first-line therapy for Raynaud's phenomenon considering their favorable long-term safety profile. These agents cause direct arterial vasodilatation.[10] A slow-release formulation is recommended for routine, long-term use.[10] However, during an acute episode of digital ischemia, the use of a short acting formulations is recommended.[10]

Phosphodiesterase-5 (PDE-5) inhibitors (sildenafil, tadalafil, vardenafil) are recommended in patients who do not satisfactorily respond to calcium channel blockers. In patients with severe attacks or critical digital ischemia, intravenous infusion of vasodilator prostaglandins, like iloprost, is advocated. This can be given during the winter months when frequent episodes

RP are expected.[10] Sympathectomy may also be considered in severe and refractory cases.[11,12]

Use of topical and systemic nitroglycerin is limited at present because of local cutaneous and systemic side effects, like headache and dizziness.[10]

DIGITAL ULCERS

Prostanoids, PDE-5 inhibitors, calcium channel blockers, and endothelin receptor antagonists (ERBs) have been recommended in the management of digital ulcers in SSc. Intravenous iloprost provides better efficacy as compared to treprostinil. However, considering the risk of side effects and the need for hospitalization, it is suggested that intravenous iloprost be administered in patients not responding to oral treatment. Intravenous iloprost combined with oral nifedipine is also beneficial. Selective PDE-5 inhibitors (tadalafil, sildenafil) are also found to be efficacious in healing and improvement of digital ulcers. The ERBs, like bosentan, are recommended in cases refractory to the above measures, especially in patients with multiple ulcers.[11] Bosentan helps in the prevention of new ulcers rather than in the healing of existing ulcers.[10]

In addition, pain and infection are to be taken care of with adequate analgesics and antibiotics. Sympathectomy may be beneficial in severe and recalcitrant cases with or without botulinum toxin injection.[12]

Management of systemic manifestations

GASTROINTESTINAL MANIFESTATIONS

The predominant gastrointestinal manifestations of SSc are pertained to gastroesophageal reflux, small intestinal bacterial overgrowth, and altered intestinal motility resulting in diarrhea or constipation.

Gastroesophageal reflux is the major common systemic symptom in these patients. Management requires modification of the patient's eating schedule; frequent small meals are recommended rather than the usual heavy ones at long intervals. Spicy and caffeine-containing food items and carbonated drinks are to be avoided. As symptomatic reflux is most common at night, the dinner can be eaten at evening hours to avoid a full stomach at bedtime. Every meal should be followed by a walk to facilitate gastric emptying. Sleeping with an elevated head and upper trunk with support minimizes the chances of reflux.

Gastroesophageal reflux is managed with proton pump inhibitors (PPIs), such as omeprazole, pantoprazole, and lansoprazole, and has been found to be effective in reducing symptoms. Long-term use of these agents is recommended, and some patients may require extra dosage.[10] The utility of PPIs in SSc-related gastroesophageal reflux is essentially based on the results extrapolated from the studies in general population as large studies to specifically evaluate their role in SSc are lacking. Antihistamines (H-2 blockers) and antacids reduce the gastric acid but are not effective in controlling reflux.[10]

Prokinetic drugs (metoclopromide, domperidone) may be used in the early stage of dysphagia or in the presence of endoscopic findings of esophagitis. A single night dose may be useful to the patient, and often long-term treatment is required. Domperidone is a better choice in this regard, because of a low side effect profile. Prokinetic agents are not useful when esophageal dysfunction is in advanced stage. Long-term use of prokinetic drugs may be associated with nutritional deficiency because of reduced absorption.[11,13–15] Hence, it is advocated that long-term use of these drugs in asymptomatic patients be discretionary.

Symptomatic small intestinal bacterial overgrowth may be treated with intermittent or rotational use of broad-spectrum antibiotics (doxycycline, quinolones, amoxicillin-clavulanate, metronidazole). However, this may predispose the patient to infection.[11,13–15]

Patients with advanced gastrointestinal disease develop malnutrition, which can be managed by oral nutritional supplementation. Parenteral nutrition should be considered when the weight loss is not corrected by enteral route. Intermittent episodes of diarrhea and constipation, which may be experienced by these patients, are managed with antidiarrheal agents and laxatives.[11,12]

Patients with SSc may experience gastric bleeding from "gastric antral vascular ectasia (GAVE)," usually managed with cryotherapy or laser photocoagulation.[10]

PULMONARY ARTERIAL HYPERTENSION

The recommendations for the management of SSc-related pulmonary arterial hypertension (PAH) are essentially in line with the management guidelines for PAH. Therapeutic decision in these patients depends upon the New York Heart Association (NYHA) functional class of the patients. The ERBs (bosentan, ambrisentan, and macitentan), selective PDE-5 inhibitors (sildenafil, tadalafil), and riociguat (a soluble guanylate cyclase stimulator) has been recommended for SSc-related PAH.

All patients of SSc with PAH are advised to maintain an active life-style. For patients with NYHA functional class I/II, an oral therapy with either of sildenafil, bosentan, or ambrisentan is started. Some authors prefer to use sildenafil at this stage because of its milder side-effects.[10] Patients who failed to respond to oral monotherapy and those with NYHA functional class III/IV should be managed with a combination therapeutic approach.[11,16] Intravenous epoprostenol has been recommended as the treatment of choice in these cases. A combination of sildenafil and bosentan may also be used, though drug interaction is a concern and there are chances of hepatotoxicity.[10] Major therapeutic alterations can be decided based on a repeat right heart catheterization.[10]

Lung or heart-lung transplantation can be considered in the case of a failure to medical therapy.[10]

SCLERODERMA RENAL CRISIS

Corticosteroids used in SSc have been shown to be significantly associated with scleroderma renal crisis (SRC), and it is recommended that SSc patients on corticosteroids be carefully and periodically monitored for any alteration in renal function and blood pressure. Other implicated risk factors include early onset diffuse SSc, anti-RNA polymerase-III antibody positivity, rapidly progressive skin sclerosis, and the presence of tendon friction rubs.

All patients with SRC must be hospitalized and closely monitored. Angiotensin converting enzyme (ACE) inhibitors (captopril, enalapril) are started immediately, and dose escalation is recommended until systolic blood pressure falls by 20 mmHg in 24 hours.[10] Initial high doses are meant for the treatment of SRC and also as a long-term therapy intending to improve renal function.[11,17] Captopril is preferred because of its faster action. If blood pressure is not controlled with a maximum dosage of ACE inhibitor, other anti-hypertensives, like calcium channel blockers, ERBs, or ARBs, can be added.[10]

Even adequate control of blood pressure may not cause reversal of the renal function and the serum creatinine level may continue to increase. Other causes of glomerular disease must be ruled out in these patients. Assessment should be based upon urinalysis (presence of red cell casts), 24-hour urinary protein excretion, and if indicated, kidney biopsy.[10] Detection of a specific pathology indicates different therapeutic approach.

In the presence of sufficient evidence that spontaneous recovery of renal function may not occur after an episode of SRC, as substantiated by renal biopsy and a recommended waiting period of six months to two years, renal transplantation may be considered.[10] This provides a better survival benefit than life-long dialysis.[10]

OTHER SYSTEMIC MANIFESTATIONS

Clinically significant cardiovascular manifestations in SSc include cardiac failure, conduction defects, and arrhythmias. In systolic heart failure, ACE inhibitors, cardioselective β-blockers, and pacemaker implantation can be considered. In diastolic failure, diuretics and calcium channel blockers are to be considered.

Musculoskeletal manifestations are benefited from the immunosuppressive therapy, and other additional symptomatic treatment is similar to that employed in general. Calcinosis cutis is an important cause of morbidity in SSc. Its management is essentially to prevent or treat any associated infection. Surgery can be considered in cases with significant morbidity affecting the quality of life.[12]

Management of cutaneous and pulmonary fibrosis

Skin and lungs are the major organs affected by fibrosis. Cutaneous fibrosis gives rise to the gradual unusual look of the patients suffering from SSc. Pulmonary involvement gives rise to interstitial lung disease (ILD). The therapy of fibrosis in SSc started with D-penicillamine, a chelating agent. However, this is out of favor at present because of high drug-related toxicity, need for prolonged monitoring, and lack of significant effectiveness in a controlled trial.[10] Anti-fibrotic therapy, effective in reversing the fibrosis in patients with SSc, is not yet in hand.

Methotrexate is recommended as a first-line treatment in early diffuse cutaneous SSc and has been associated with significant improvement in skin thickness scores. The usual dosage employed has been in the range of 15 mg/week and a dosage of 25 mg/m[2] in the pediatric age group. No data, however, is available showing the higher doses (as in rheumatoid arthritis) offer any significant benefit. Azathioprine and mycophenolate mofetil have also been used for skin sclerosis in SSc.[11]

Cyclophosphamide is recommended for ILD, especially in the progressive form. Administered at a dose of 1–2 mg/kg/day, cyclophosphamide was shown to improve dyspnea, lung volume, high resolution computed tomography scores, and quality of life. The lung functions continued to improve after cessation of therapy as well for up to six months. It is, however, recommended that the dosage and duration of cyclophosphamide be individualized based on the extent and severity of the disease at presentation and response to treatment. Either of the daily oral dose or monthly intravenous dose may be administered.[10] Long-term maintenance therapy or sequential therapy with other immunosuppressive drugs may be required for a persistent therapeutic response.[10] Cyclophosphamide has been shown to improve the skin manifestations as well.[11,18,19] Mycophenolate mofetil is considered as an alternative to cyclophosphamide.[10]

A couple of randomized controlled trials have shown greater beneficial effects of autologous hematopoietic stem cell therapy (HSCT) with immunosuppression as compared to cyclophosphamide alone in the treatment of skin and lung disease. Because of the therapy-related adverse effects and early therapy-related mortality associated with HSCT, it must be considered carefully in selected patients with rapidly progressive disease and risk of organ failure.[11,20,21]

Various agents preventing the pro-fibrotic pathways involved in the pathogenesis of SSc have been tried in the treatment of fibrosis in patients with SSc.[10] A human recombinant antibody targeting transforming growth factor-β (TGF-β) versus placebo has been tried in early diffuse SSc, without significant effect on skin score and lung function tests.[10] Various tyrosine kinase inhibitors and platelet-derived growth factor (PDGF)-inhibitors (imatinib, dasatinib, nilotinib) have demonstrated anti-fibrotic effects in *in vitro* studies and animal models; however, efficacy of these agents have not been proved in uncontrolled trials.[10]

REFERENCES

1. Careta MF, Romiti R. Localized scleroderma: Clinical spectrum and therapeutic update. *An Bras Dermatol* 2015;90:62–73.
2. Kroft EB, Groeneveld TJ, Seyger MM, de Jong EM. Efficacy of topical tacrolimus 0.1% in active plaque morphea: Randomized, double-blind, emolient-controlled pilot study. *Am J Clin Dermatol* 2009;10:181–187.
3. Campione E, Paterno EJ, Diluvio L, Orlandi A, Bianchi L, Chimenti S. Localized morphea treated with imiquimod 5% and dermoscopic assessment of effectiveness. *J Dermatolog Treat* 2009;20:10–13.
4. Dytoc MT, Kossintseva I, Ting PT. First case series on the use of calcipotriol-betamethasone dipropionate for morphea. *Br J Dermatol* 2007;157:615–618.
5. Kreuter A, Gambichler T, Avermaete A et al. Combined treatment with calcipotriol ointment and low-dose ultraviolet A I phototherapy in childhood morphea. *Pediatr Dermatol* 2001;18:241–245.
6. Li SC, Torok KS, Pope E et al. Development of consensus treatment plans for juvenile localized scleroderma: A roadmap toward comparative effectiveness studies in juvenile localized scleroderma. *Arthritis Care Res (Hoboken)* 2012;64:1175–1185.
7. Martini G, Ramanan AV, Falcini F, Girschick H, Goldsmith DP, Zulian F. Successful treatment of severe or methotrexate resistant juvenile localized scleroderma with mycophenolate mofetil. *Rheumatology (Oxford)* 2009;48:1410–1413.
8. Diab M, Coloe JR, Magro C, Bechtel MA. Treatment of recalcitrant generalized morphea with infliximab. *Arch Dermatol* 2010;146:601–604.
9. Moinzadeh P, Krieg T, Hunzelmann N. Imatinib treatment of generalized localized scleroderma (morphea). *J Am Acad Dermatol* 2010;63:e102–e104.
10. Boin F, Wigley FM. Clinical features and treatment of scleroderma. In: Firestein GS, Budd RC, Gabriel SE, McInnes IB,

O'Dell JR, Eds. *Kelley's Textbook of Rheumatology*, Vol. 2, 9th ed. Philadelphia, PA: Elsevier Saunders, 2013, pp. 1363–1403.

11. Kowal-Bielecka O, Fransen J, Avouac J et al. Update of EULAR recommendations for the treatment of systemic sclerosis. *Ann Rheum Dis* 2017;76:1327–1339.

12. Denton CP, Hughes M, Gak N et al. BSR and BHPR guideline for the treatment of systemic sclerosis. *Rheumatology (Oxford)* 2016;55:1906–1910.

13. Donnellan C, Sharma N, Preston C, Moayyedi P. Medical treatments for the maintenance therapy of reflux oesopha-gitis and endoscopic negative reflux disease. *Cochrane Database Syst Rev* 2005;(2):CD003245.

14. Sigterman KE, van Pinxteren B, Bonis PA, Lau J, Numans ME. Short-term treatment with proton pump inhibitors, H2-receptor antago-nists and prokinetics for gastro-oesophageal reflux disease-like symptoms and endoscopy negative reflux disease. *Cochrane Database Syst Rev* 2013;5:CD002095.

15. Ali T, Roberts DN, Tierney WM. Long-term safety concerns with proton pump inhibi-tors. *Am J Med* 2009;122:896–903.

16. Galiè N, Humbert M, Vachiery JL et al. 2015 ESC/ERS guidelines for the diagnosis and treatment of pulmonary hypertension: The Joint Task Force for the Diagnosis and Treatment of Pulmonary Hypertension of the European Society of Cardiology (ESC) and the European Respiratory Society (ERS): Endorsed by: Association for European Paediatric and Congenital Cardiology (AEPC), International Society for Heart and Lung Transplantation (ISHLT). *Eur Heart J* 2016;37:67–119.

17. Khanna D. Diagnosis and management of systemic sclerosis. *Indian J Rheumatol* 2010;5:69–75.

18. Tashkin DP, Elashoff R, Clements PJ et al. Cyclophosphamide versus placebo in scleroderma lung disease. *N Engl J Med* 2006;354:2655–2666.

19. Goldin J, Elashoff R, Kim HJ et al. Treatment of scleroderma-interstitial lung disease with cyclophosphamide is associated with less progressive fibrosis on serial thoracic high-resolution CT scan than placebo: Findings from the scleroderma lung study. *Chest* 2009;136:1333–1340.

20. Burt RK, Shah SJ, Dill K et al. Autologous non-myeloablative haemopoietic stem-cell transplantation compared with pulse cyclophosphamide once per month for systemic sclerosis (ASSIST): An open-label, randomised phase 2 trial. *Lancet* 2011;378:498–506.

21. van Laar JM, Farge D, Sont JK et al. Autologous hematopoietic stem cell trans-plantation vs intravenous pulse cyclophos-phamide in diffuse cutaneous systemic sclerosis: A randomized clinical trial. *JAMA* 2014;311:2490–2498.

7

Scleroderma overlap syndromes

AKANKSHA KAUSHIK AND M. SENDHIL KUMARAN

INTRODUCTION

Scleroderma, or systemic sclerosis (SSc), is a collagen vascular disorder characterized by immune dysregulation, widespread tissue fibrosis and sclerosis of skin (Figure 7.1). Two main subtypes of SSc include limited cutaneous (lSSc) and diffuse cutaneous (dSSc).

The term "autoimmunity kaleidoscope" was coined by Hudson et al (2008). with reference to scleroderma patients, pertaining to two or more autoimmune diseases co-existing in a single patient (polyautoimmunity), or in the same household; this phenomenon is designated as polyautoimmunity or familial autoimmunity respectively.[1] Patients with scleroderma are often found to have co-existing features of other collagen vascular disorders and are designated as "overlap syndromes."

Overlap syndrome is a condition in which the diagnostic criteria of at least two collagen vascular disorders is satisfied.[2] Many collagen vascular disorders may co-exist, precede, or even follow the onset of scleroderma. Such patients are categorized as scleroderma overlap syndrome. The collagen vascular disorders reported to co-exist with scleroderma include:

- Inflammatory myositis, like polymyositis/dermatomyositis (PM/DM)
- Sjögren syndrome (SS)
- Systemic lupus erythematosus (SLE)
- Rheumatoid arthritis (RA)
- Antiphospholipid antibody (APLA) syndrome
- Others (including sarcoidosis, vasculitis, and autoimmune hepatitis)

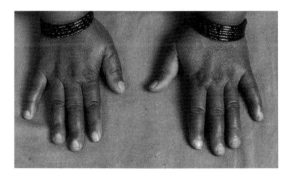

Figure 7.1 Acral sclerosis in a patient with SSc.

EPIDEMIOLOGY

The frequency of scleroderma overlap syndrome ranges from 10% to 38%, as recorded in multiple cohort studies.[1,3,4] Females manifest overlap syndrome more frequently than males. As compared to patients with scleroderma, those having scleroderma overlap syndrome are more often found to have a positive family history for rheumatological disorders; they have had more frequent use of corticosteroids and immunosuppressives as therapeutic agents as well.

Scleroderma overlap with inflammatory myositis (PM/DM) has been reported to be one of the most common overlap syndromes in many cohort studies. One of these studies reported musculoskeletal involvement being as high as 62.5%.[4] Other common overlap syndromes include Scleroderma-Sjögren's syndrome (SSc/SS) overlap (reported incidence 16.8%–42.5%) and Scleroderma-Rheumatoid arthritis (SSc/RA) overlap (incidence 4.6%–32%).[5] Scleroderma and Systemic lupus erythematosus (SSc/SLE) overlap is seen in about 8% cases. Anti-phospholipid antibodies have been reported in 7%–13% of scleroderma patients, even though all manifestations of APLA syndrome may not be manifested. Among hepatic autoimmune disorders, scleroderma overlap has been described with primary biliary cirrhosis (PBC). In PBC, the prevalence of SSc is up to 15%, and most of them are associated with the lSSc subtype. Sarcoidosis, thyroid disorders, and celiac disease constitute other rare entities reported with scleroderma. Most patients with scleroderma overlap syndrome are younger in age, as compared to individual collagen vascular disorders, particularly the SSc/SLE overlap syndrome.[6]

CLINICAL AND IMMUNE SPECTRUM

Scleroderma and inflammatory myositis

Myositis may appear before, after, or simultaneously with the onset of scleroderma. The diffuse cutaneous form is the predominant form associated with myositis and association with cardiomyopathy has been reported. Gut involvement and related complications like pneumatosis intestinalis and pseudo-obstruction have been commonly reported. Studies have reported SSc/myositis overlap to be associated with specific autoantibodies like anti-PM-Scl, anti-U2 RNP, anti-Ku, and anti-U5 snRNP. Occurrence of anti-PM-Scl antibodies parallels with arthritis, and the course of interstitial lung disease (ILD) with this association is benign. Anti-Jo-1 antibodies are not commonly seen. Scleroderma/myositis overlap syndrome is considered a severe form with reported mortality rate as high as 21%.

Scleroderma and Sjögren's syndrome

Patients with SSc/SS overlap syndrome mainly have localized cutaneous subtype of scleroderma and a lower frequency of lung fibrosis. Appearance of anti-centromere antibody (ACA) precedes the development of scleroderma by several years in patients with Sjögren's syndrome. In SSc/SS overlap syndrome, co-existence with PBC has also been described. Baldini et al (2013). have reported mild organ involvement but increased risk of non-Hodgkin's lymphomas (NHLs) in ACA-positive overlap of lcSSc and Sjögren's syndrome.[7]

Scleroderma and systemic lupus erythematosus

Scleroderma/SLE overlap has been reported frequently. SSc/SLE overlap runs a progressively fatal course and even a grave outcome. Features like pulmonary arterial hypertension (PAH), pancreatitis, polyserositis, avascular necrosis of bone, and leukoencephalopathy have been described. This overlap syndrome shows high titers of anti-double stranded DNA (anti-dsDNA) and anti-PM/Scl. Rare cases of shrinking lung syndrome have also been described in this overlap syndrome.[8]

In the case of dermatological presentation of overlap syndromes, particularly those of scleroderma and SLE, a "dermatologic classification of overlap syndromes" has been proposed as presented in Table 7.1.[9]

Scleroderma and rheumatoid arthritis

Scleroderma may develop in long-standing rheumatoid arthritis (RA), and conversely, established dSSc patients may develop rheumatoid factor (RF) positive RA; this is especially in scleroderma associated with interstitial lung disease (ILD) and scl-70 antibodies. Mostly, the

Table 7.1 Dermatologic classification of overlap syndromes

Type 1	Systemic disease overlapping with systemic disease
Type 2	Cutaneous disease (e.g., localized scleroderma, cutaneous LE) overlapping with systemic disease (e.g., systemic LE)
Type 3	Cutaneous disease (e.g., localized scleroderma) overlapping with cutaneous disease (e.g., cutaneous LE); overlap may occur with distinctive lesions developing at separate sites or clinical and/or histological features of both diseases within the same site (known as coincident overlap)

onset of SSc precedes that of RA.[10] Both SSc- and RA-associated HLA-DR alleles have been detected in SSc-RA overlap. RF and anti-cyclic citrullinated peptide (CCP) antibodies occur in between 25% and 10.6% of the SSc patients, respectively. In SSc, presence of anti-CCP2 antibodies strongly correlate with arthritis and a radiological feature of marginal erosions. Overall, the anti-CCP antibody titers are lower in SSc/RA overlap as compared to RA alone.

Scleroderma and Antiphospholipid Antibody syndrome

Although anti beta-2-glycoprotein-1 antibodies (lupus anticoagulant) have not been reported, it may be present in scleroderma. These cases may be complicated with pulmonary arterial hypertension (PAH), peripheral ischemia (Figure 7.2), hemolytic-uremic syndrome, glomerular thrombosis, myocardial ischemia, and thrombo-embolism. Death may be a sequel in presence of any of these complications.

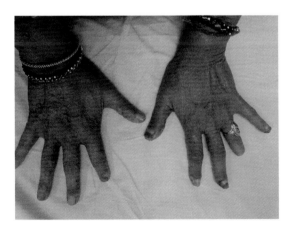

Figure 7.2 Peripheral ischemia leading to gangrene and amputation of a digit.

Scleroderma and other conditions

- **Scleroderma and sarcoidosis:** This overlap is rare. Presence of fever, weight loss, and hilar lymphadenopathy indicates the possibility of sarcoidosis in a patient with scleroderma. Testing for angiotensin-converting enzyme (ACE) is not useful; biopsy from lymph nodes may be helpful in these patients.
- **Scleroderma and liver diseases:** Overlap between scleroderma and primary biliary cirrhosis (PBC) has been described. PBC mostly seems to occur in localized cutaneous scleroderma and is usually silent, despite elevation in cholestatic enzymes and anti-mitochondrial antibodies. Anti-centromere antibody (ACA) is a useful marker in these patients. Positive ACA in PBC seems to predict a future risk of scleroderma. The incidence of positive ACA is higher in SSc/PBC overlap than in SSc alone. The three major antigenic polypeptides recognized by ACA are CENP-A, CENP-B, and CENP-C; increased reactivity to CENP-C has been reported in PBC/CREST overlap syndrome. The anti-myositis antibody (AMA) positivity is also frequent, although non-specific. However, the pathogenic role for these antibodies has not been proved. Other liver diseases in scleroderma are extremely uncommon; autoimmune hepatitis and sclerosing cholangitis have been reported rarely.
- **Scleroderma and thyroid diseases:** Thyroid diseases like hypothyroidism and Grave's disease have been reported to occur in scleroderma (13% and 2.5%, respectively). Scleroderma patients with anti-thyroid peroxidase (TPO) antibodies carry the risk of developing thyroid dysfunction.
- **Scleroderma and celiac disease:** Celiac disease has been rarely reported in women with a localized cutaneous form of scleroderma.

DIAGNOSIS

Diagnosis of overlap syndrome is made in the presence of the diagnostic criteria of at least two connective tissue diseases.

Clinical suspicion should arise based upon the clinical presentation. Most scleroderma overlap syndromes have an associated typical antibody profile, although not diagnostic, can provide useful clues in identifying the underlying syndrome. These are summarized in Table 7.2.

Additional tests should be done based upon the clinical features of a given patient; e.g., in a patient with features of scleroderma and muscle pain, serum creatinine phosphokinase (CPK) should be done. In established myositis, chest radiography and spirometry, along with high-resolution computerized tomographic scan (HR-CT) are to be done. In patients presenting with features of congestive cardiac failure, evaluation for cardiac enzymes and/or MRI can be done. Recently, Elessawy et al (2016). have reported the usefulness of whole-body MRI in detecting muscle and subcutaneous edema as markers of perivascular inflammation in patients with myositis, including those having SSc-myositis overlap.[11]

The diagnosis of scleroderma overlap syndrome rests upon diagnosing scleroderma by the American College of Rheumatology/European League Against Rheumatism (ACR/EULAR) criteria (2013)[12] presented in Chapter 4. Scleroderma can then be sub-divided into limited cutaneous or diffuse cutaneous subtypes by the classification system proposed by LeRoy et al.[13]

Summary of the currently followed clinical criteria for diagnosing overlap syndromes are presented in Table 7.3. Diagnosis of other rare overlap syndromes is made on the basis of clinical presentation and associated antibodies.

INVESTIGATIONS ON FOLLOW UP

As in connective tissue disorders, acute phase reactants may be elevated in acute flares but their role in scleroderma overlap syndromes has not been studied. Scoring systems like the modified Rodnan skin score (mRSS), which are widely used in dSSc to measure skin thickness and disease activity,[14] have not been used in specific studies pertaining to scleroderma overlap. Investigations like ultrasonographic measurement of skin thickness and elastometry have similarly not been studied and still do not have a definite role in overlap syndromes.

Low-serum complement levels (C3 and C4) is a potential marker of disease activity in SSc overlap syndromes. In a large cohort study in 321 patients with systemic sclerosis, Hudson et al (2007). suggested that hypocomplementemia is significantly more common in SSc overlap syndromes than pure SSc.[15] Recently, Esposito et al (2016). have reported that hypocomplementemia is associated with SSc overlap syndrome, especially SSc-PM overlap, and is a useful marker to monitor disease activity and response to therapy.[16]

In patients with evidence of interstitial lung disease, pulmonary function tests (PFT) may be needed at baseline diagnosis and followed by annual tests as needed, although no recommendations specifically for scleroderma overlap syndrome have been made.

MANAGEMENT

Management of scleroderma overlap syndrome is not standardized, mainly due to the absence of controlled trials. Management strategies are based upon conventional therapies followed for individual collagen vascular disorders.

Table 7.2 Scleroderma overlap syndromes and related serological profile

Scleroderma overlap syndrome	Antibodies
SSc/Myositis overlap	Anti-PM-Scl, anti-U2 RNP, anti-Ku, anti-U5 snRNP, anti-Mi2
SSc/Sjögren syndrome overlap	Anti-Ro 52, anti-nRNP
SSc/RA overlap	ANA, IgM RF, anti-CCP antibodies (mostly anti-CCP2)
SSc/SLE overlap	Anti-double stranded DNA (Anti-dsDNA), anti-PM/Scl.
SSc/PBC overlap	Anti-centromere antibody (ACA), AMA (less specific)
SSc/APLA syndrome overlap	Anti-β- 2-glycoprotein-1
SSc-Thyroid disease overlap	Anti-TPO antibodies

Table 7.3 Diagnosis of some of the common scleroderma overlap syndromes

Diagnosis	Clinical and laboratory criteria
Scleroderma–PM overlap syndrome	Muscle weakness with elevated creatinine kinase (CK) and two of the following: (1) Inflammatory myositis from muscle biopsy (2) Abnormal electromyography (EMG) (3) Positive for anti-PM-Scl or anti-Ku
Scleroderma–Dermatomyositis overlap syndrome	Dermatomyositis skin lesions (i.e., heliotrope, Gottron's sign, Gottron's papule) plus three of the following: (1) Muscle weakness (2) Elevated CK (3) Inflammatory myositis from muscle biopsy (4) Abnormal electromyography (EMG) (5) Positive for anti-Mi2
Scleroderma–SLE overlap syndrome	Four or more of the following criteria with at least one clinical and one laboratory criteria according to Systemic Lupus International Collaborating Clinics (SLICC) Classification Criteria 2012 for SLE or kidney biopsy proven-lupus nephritis with ANA or anti-dsDNA positive: Clinical criteria composed of: (1) Acute cutaneous lupus (2) Chronic cutaneous lupus (3) Oral or nasal ulcers (4) Non-scarring alopecia (5) Arthritis (6) Serositis (7) Renal involvement (8) Neurological involvement (9) Hemolytic anemia (10) Leukopenia (11) Thrombocytopenia Laboratory criteria composed of (1) ANA (2) Anti-dsDNA (3) Anti-Sm (4) Antiphospholipid antibodies (5) Low complement (6) Direct Coombs' test in the absence of hemolytic anemia

(Continued)

Table 7.3 (*Continued*) Diagnosis of some of the common scleroderma overlap syndromes

Diagnosis	Clinical and laboratory criteria
Scleroderma-RA overlap syndrome	Total score ≥6 according to 2010 ACR-EULAR classification criteria for RA: Joint distribution (1) 1 large joint (score = 0) (2) 2–10 large joints (score = 1) (3) 1–3 small joints (score = 2) (4) 4–10 small joints (score = 3) (5) >10 joints (score = 5) Serology (1) Negative RF and negative anti-CCP (score = 0) (2) Low positive RF or low positive anti-CCP (score = 2) (3) High positive RF or high positive anti-CCP (score = 3) Duration of symptoms (1) <6 weeks (score = 0) (2) ≥6 weeks (score = 1) Acute phase reactants (1) Normal CRP and normal ESR (score = 0) (2) High CRP or high ESR (score = 1)
Scleroderma–PM–SLE overlap syndrome	PM plus clinical features of SLE and the specific serology for PM or SLE

Source: Foocharoen, C. et al., *Int. J. Rheum. Dis.*, 19, 913–923, 2016.

Many clinical features in overlap syndromes are intermittent, non-debilitating and are highly responsive to steroids (e.g., myositis, pleurisy, pericarditis, and myocarditis). Severe systemic complications like nephrotic syndrome, Raynaud's phenomenon and deforming arthropathy do not respond well to corticosteroids. Many of the typical scleroderma-associated manifestations in overlap syndromes can be managed on the same lines as primary scleroderma, e.g., angiotensin-converting enzyme (ACE) inhibitors for renal crisis, calcium channel blockers for Raynaud's phenomenon, and proton pump inhibitors for dyspepsia and heartburn.

However, fibrotic lung disease and alveolitis is mostly resistant to prednisolone and commonly used immunosuppressive agents. Some studies suggest that tyrosine kinase inhibitors (e.g., imatinib) may be effective in these patients.[17] Table 7.4 summarizes various clinical scenario-based common therapeutic modalities in overlap syndromes.

Concerns during therapy of specific scleroderma overlap syndromes

- *Scleroderma myositis overlap*: In scleroderma-myositis overlap, treatment is mainly directed against the alveolitis, muscle, and skin damage. Corticosteroids and adjuvant immunosuppressive drugs like methotrexate, azathioprine, mycophenolate mofetil, and cyclophosphamide are commonly used. Although high-dose systemic steroids are effective in myositis, they may provoke renal crisis in patients with dSSc; hence, special caution and monitoring is required.

  Reduction in steroid dosage may be achieved with the use of antitumor necrosis factor (TNF) alpha antibodies like infliximab, which has recently been reported to produce significant improvement in debilitating calcinosis in scleroderma-myositis overlap.[18] However, anti-TNF alpha agents may worsen

Table 7.4 Summary of common treatment modalities in overlap syndromes

Manifestation	Treatment
Non-specific constitutional features, e.g., fever, fatigue, myalgias, arthralgias	Non-steroidal anti-inflammatory drugs (NSAID), anti-malarials, low-dose prednisolone (<10 mg/day) Trial use of modafinil
Vascular headache	Trial of propranolol and/or alternate-day aspirin, 350 mg Symptomatic use of a triptan (e.g., sumatriptin, eletriptan)
Autoimmune anemia and thrombocytopenia	High dose steroids (prednisolone, ~80 mg/day) gradually tapered depending upon clinical course. Consider danazol, intravenous immunoglobulin G (IVIG), and immunosuppressives in recalcitrant cases.
Thrombotic thrombocytopenic purpura	Immediate infusion of fresh frozen plasma. May require plasma exchange and transfusion of platelet depleted RBCs. Consider splenectomy in recalcitrant cases
Raynaud's phenomenon	Keep extremities warm, avoid finger trauma, avoid β-blockers, stop smoking. Dihydropyridine, Ca- channel blockers (e.g., nifedipine). Alpha sympatholytics (e.g., prazosin). Consider endothelin receptor antagonist (e.g., bosentan) in recalcitrant cases
Acute-onset digital gangrene	Local chemical sympathectomy (infiltration of lidocaine at the base of involved digit). Anti-coagulation, Topical nitrates, Consider hospitalization for intra-arterial prostacyclin. Start endothelin receptor antagonist therapy. Consider hyperbaric oxygen
Arthritis	NSAIDs, anti-malarials, methotrexate, consider tumor necrosis factor (TNF) inhibitors in severe cases.
Pulmonary arterial hypertension (PAH)	Trial of steroids, cyclophosphamide and low dose aspirin in asymptomatic PAH. In symptomatic PAH, intravenous prostacyclin, ACE inhibitors, bosentan, anti-coagulation
Scleroderma-like renal crisis	ACE inhibitors
Membranous nephropathy and nephrotic syndrome	Steroids are useful but not fully effective. ACE inhibitors reduce proteinuria. Low dose aspirin and dipyridamole reduce thrombotic complications. Severe cases require pulse cyclophosphamide and trial of Rituximab
Cardiac complications	Prednisolone and NSAIDs in pericarditis; Prednisolone and/or cyclophosphamide in myocarditis. Digoxin is contraindicated.

(Continued)

Table 7.4 (*Continued*) Summary of common treatment modalities in overlap syndromes

Manifestation	Treatment
Dysphagia	Mild—no treatment
	With reflux—proton pump inhibitor. Consider Nissen fundoplication
	Severe—Calcium channel antagonist, alone or in combination with an anti-cholinergic agent
	Prokinetics like metoclopromide may be used in intestinal dysmotility
Heartburn/reflux	Raise head end of bed, discontinue smoking, lose weight, and avoid caffeine. H2- antagonists, H^+ proton pump blockers. Metoclopramide use is under trial. Consider management of *H. Pylori* infection in recalcitrant cases
Myositis	Acute onset/severe: prednisolone, 60–100 mg/day
	Chronic/low grade: prednisolone, 10–30 mg/day
	Consider methotrexate and/or IVIG in recalcitrant cases
Osteoporosis	Calcium/Vitamin D supplements, estrogen replacement, or raloxifene. Biphosphonates. Nasal calcitonin. Carboxyl truncated PTH analogs such as hPTH

interstitial lung disease (ILD) and alveolitis; hence, the use of these agents has to be individualized.

Effective treatment of myositis, joint, or skin disease may not equally control the underlying alveolitis in these patients. Alveolitis is also a relative contraindication for the use of methotrexate. IVIG and mycophenolate mofetil have been reported to improve skin and muscle involvement, as well as alveolitis and gut complications.[19–21] Eculizumab has been recently used successfully in scleroderma renal crisis in SSc/myositis overlap.[22]

- *Scleroderma-Sjögren syndrome overlap:* Use of anti-TNF alpha agents have produced mixed results. Rituximab has shown efficacy in control of systemic features.
- *Scleroderma-RA overlap:* Initial therapy involves the use of NSAIDs, aspirin, and DMARDs. Safety issues are a concern with the use of anti-TNF therapy for joint involvement in SSc/RA overlap. There are reports of scleroderma-like changes with the use of infliximab, as well as fatal pneumonitis with the use of adalimumab in these patients. Since

CD20+ B-lymphocytes have been reported in scleroderma lesions and raised interleukin-6 (IL-6) levels have been documented in this category of overlap syndromes, rituximab (anti-CD20 antibody), and tocilizumab (anti-IL-6 receptor antibody) may be useful.

- *Scleroderma-SLE overlap:* Overlap of SSc/SLE has treatment implications as well. In SSc/SLE patients who develop renal failure and hypertension, it is essential to distinguish between lupus nephritis and scleroderma renal crisis. Concomitant dSSc may limit the use of steroids in SLE, whereas flares of SLE may limit the use of anti-TNF alpha agents in SSc.[23] Rituximab and mycophenolate mofetil have been found to be safe and efficacious agents in the management of SSc/SLE overlap syndrome.

NATURAL COURSE

The natural course and prognosis of overlap syndromes is variable and depends upon the individual patient, response to therapy, as well as the underlying pathology. SSc-myositis overlap with anti-PM/Scl positivity generally have mild myositis and show good response to corticosteroids.[24] However, a small fraction of SSc-myositis patients who are positive for Scl-70 generally have a higher mortality and morbidity than pure scleroderma. Baldini et al. have reported that patients with SSc/SS overlap with positive anticentromere antibody (ACA) are at a higher risk of lymphomas, although the systemic features may be mild.[7] Higher anti-CCP2 titers in SSc/RA overlap are related to greater arthritis and marginal erosions on X-ray.[25] Raised IL-6 levels in SSc/RA overlap correlate with increased severity of skin and lung fibrosis as well as pulmonary arterial hypertension.

REFERENCES

1. Hudson M, Rojas-Villarraga A, Coral-Alvarado P et al. Polyautoimmunity and familial autoimmunity in systemic sclerosis. *J Autoimmun* 2008;31:156–159.
2. Rodriguez-Reyna TS, Alarcon-Segovia D. Overlap syndromes in the context of shared autoimmunity. *Autoimmunity* 2005;38:219–223.
3. Caramaschi P, Biasi D, Volpe A, Carletto A, Cecchetto M, Bambara LM. Coexistence of systemic sclerosis with other autoimmune diseases. *Rheumatol Int* 2007;27:407–410.
4. Moinzadeh P, Aberer E, Ahmadi-Simab K et al. Disease progression in systemic sclerosis-overlap syndrome is significantly different from limited and diffuse cutaneous systemic sclerosis. *Ann Rheum Dis* 2015;74:730–737.
5. Pakozdi A, Nihtyanova S, Moinzadeh P, Ong VH, Black CM, Denton CP. Clinical and serological hallmarks of systemic sclerosis overlap syndromes. *J Rheumatol* 2011;38:2406–2409.
6. Foocharoen C, Netwijitpan S, Mahakkanukrauh A, Suwannaroj S, Nanagara R. Clinical characteristics of scleroderma overlap syndromes: Comparisons with pure scleroderma. *Int J Rheum Dis* 2016;19:913–923.
7. Baldini C, Mosca M, Della Rossa A et al. Overlap of ACA-positive systemic sclerosis and Sjögren's syndrome: A distinct clinical entity with mild organ involvement but at high risk of lymphoma. *Clin Exp Rheumatol* 2013;31:272–280.
8. Guleria VS, Singh PK, Saxena P, Subramanian S. Shrinking lung syndrome in systemic lupus erythematosus-scleroderma overlap. *Lung India* 2014;31:407–409.
9. Pascucci A, Lynch PJ, Fazel N. Lupus erythematosus and localized scleroderma coexistent at the same sites: A rare presentation of overlap syndrome of connective-tissue diseases. *Cutis* 2016;97:359–363.
10. Szucs G, Szekanecz Z, Zilahi E et al. Systemic sclerosis-rheumatoid arthritis overlap syndrome: A unique combination of features suggests a distinct genetic, serological and clinical entity. *Rheumatology (Oxford)* 2007;46:989–993.
11. Elessawy SS, Abdelsalam EM, Abdel Razek E, Tharwat S. Whole-body MRI for full assessment and characterization of diffuse inflammatory myopathy. *Acta Radiol Open* 2016;5:2058460116668216.
12. LeRoy EC, Black C, Fleischmajer R et al. Scleroderma (systemic sclerosis): Classification, subsets and pathogenesis. *J Rheumatol* 1988;15:202–205.
13. van den Hoogen F, Khanna D, Fransen J et al. 2013 classification criteria for systemic sclerosis: An American College of Rheumatology/European League against Rheumatism collaborative initiative. *Arthritis Rheum* 2013;65:2737–2747.
14. Hurwitz EL, Wong WK, Seibold JR et al. Skin thickness score as a predictor and correlate of outcome in systemic sclerosis: High-dose versus low-dose penicillamine trial. *Arthritis Rheum* 2000;43:2445–2454.
15. Hudson M, Walker JG, Fritzler M, Taillefer S, Baron M. Hypocomplementemia in systemic sclerosis—Clinical and serological correlations. *J Rheumatol* 2007;34:2218–2223.
16. Esposito J, Brown Z, Stevens W et al. The association of low complement with disease activity in systemic sclerosis: A prospective cohort study. *Arthritis Res Ther* 2016;18:246.
17. Distler JH, Distler O. Tyrosine kinase inhibitors for the treatment of fibrotic diseases such as systemic sclerosis: Towards molecular targeted therapies. *Ann Rheum Dis* 2010;69 Suppl 1:i48–i51.

18. Tosounidou S, MacDonald H, Situnayake D. Successful treatment of calcinosis with infliximab in a patient with systemic sclerosis/myositis overlap syndrome. *Rheumatology (Oxford)* 2014;53:960–961.
19. Levy Y, Amital H, Langevitz P et al. Intravenous immunoglobulin modulates cutaneous involvement and reduces skin fibrosis in systemic sclerosis: An open-label study. *Arthritis Rheum* 2004;50:1005–1007.
20. Nihtyanova SI, Brough GM, Black CM, Denton CP. Mycophenolate mofetil in diffuse cutaneous systemic sclerosis—A retrospective analysis. *Rheumatology (Oxford)*. 2007;46:442–445.
21. Abelha-Aleixo J, Bernardo A, Costa L. Benefit of intravenous immunoglobulin in a patient with longstanding polymyositis/systemic sclerosis overlap syndrome. *Acta Reumatol Port* 2015;40:176–178.
22. Thomas CP, Nester CM, Phan AC, Sharma M, Steele AL, Lenert PS. Eculizumab for rescue of thrombotic microangiopathy in PM-Scl antibody-positive autoimmune overlap syndrome. *Clin Kidney J* 2015;8:698–701.
23. Christopher-Stine L, Wigley F. Tumor necrosis factor-alpha antagonists induce lupus-like syndrome in patients with scleroderma overlap/mixed connective tissue disease. *J Rheumatol* 2003;30:2725–2727.
24. Jablonska S, Blaszyk M. Scleromyositis (scleroderma/polymyositis overlap) is an entity. *J Eur Acad Dermatol Venereol* 2004;18:265–266.
25. Ingegnoli F, Galbiati V, Zeni S et al. Use of antibodies recognizing cyclic citrullinated peptide in the differential diagnosis of joint involvement in systemic sclerosis. *Clin Rheumatol* 2007;26:510–514.

8

Childhood scleroderma

MUHAMMED RAZMI T. AND RAHUL MAHAJAN

INTRODUCTION

Pediatric scleroderma includes localized scleroderma (LSc) and juvenile systemic sclerosis (JSSc). The predominant form of childhood scleroderma is LSc, also known as morphea, which principally involves the skin and underlying musculoskeletal structures. JSSc is a chronic, multisystem, collagen vascular disorder characterized by symmetrical fibrous thickening and hardening of the skin combined with similar fibrotic changes in the major organs. JSSc has been classified based on the extent of skin and the associated internal organ involvement. LSc and JSSc with limited cutaneous involvement (lSSc) are distinct entities; while LSc has been restricted to involve cutaneous structures almost exclusively, JSSc tends to involve internal organs.

LOCALIZED SCLERODERMA

Localized scleroderma affects almost exclusively the skin with some involvement of underlying musculature without any internal organ involvement. However, in extremely rare cases, these patients may develop some extra-cutaneous manifestations during the course of the disease. Owing to the localized involvement of the disease, the major complications in untreated patients are due to the deformities of the affected areas without any impact on the longevity.

Various classifications have been proposed for LSc. The one proposed by Laxer and Zulian (2006) has been followed here. According to this classification, LSc has been identified as five subtypes, namely circumscribed (plaque) morphea, generalized morphea, linear morphea, pansclerotic morphea, and mixed morphea.

Epidemiology

In a large, retrospective, multicenter review of 750 children with LSc, the most common subtype was linear morphea (65%), followed by circumscribed morphea (26%), generalized morphea (7%), and deep morphea (2%). An overlap of different types of morphea (mixed morphea) was noted in 12%.[1]

Clinical features

CIRCUMSCRIBED (PLAQUE) MORPHEA

This is the most benign form of morphea. There are single or few discrete, erythematous, oval, or round plaques usually confined to a single anatomic area. In the early active phase, the lesion is erythematous and shows a "lilac hue" at the periphery (Figure 8.1). This is followed by an indurated phase with progressive dermal thickening as evidenced by sclerosis and central atrophy. During the course of the disease, the lesions become atrophic and sometimes hypopigmented. Often there is self-resolution after 3–5 years (Figure 8.2). In this variant of morphea, the major brunt of the disease process is in the dermis with minimal involvement of the subcutaneous tissue.

Several variants of this entity have been described. *Guttate morphea* resembles lichen sclerosus *et* atrophicus, except for the hyperpigmented healing phase. Multiple subcentimetric erythematous to hypopigmented papules with minimal sclerosis affect frequently the trunk in guttate morphea (Figure 8.3). *Keloidal* or *nodular morphea* is characterized by the occurrence of keloid-like nodules in association with previous or co-existent morphea, or SSc. Histopathology may show features

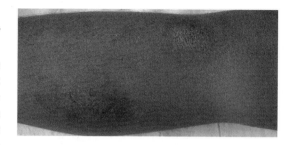

Figure 8.2 Residual lesion of morphea following resolution.

of morphea with keloidal collagen. *Atrophoderma of Pasini and Pierini* is rare in children and usually affects adolescents and young adults. In this variant, atrophic but non-indurated, hyper-pigmented or skin-colored symmetrical plaques can be seen on the trunks with sharply defined "cliff-drop" border. *Morphea profunda* and *subcutaneous morphea* are characterized by fibrosis involving the deeper subcutaneous tissue and muscles.

GENERALIZED MORPHEA

It is defined as the presence of ≥4 plaques of ≥3 cm size involving ≥2 out of 7 different anatomical sites (head–neck, right-upper extremity, left-upper extremity, right-lower extremity, left-lower extremity, anterior trunk, posterior trunk). Usually, the trunk and limbs are involved. The disease process is severe and rapidly progressive. Generalized morphea accounts for up to 10% of pediatric cases, while it is up to 50% in adults. Constitutional symptoms like myalgia, arthralgia, and fatigue are common, and extra-cutaneous manifestations like dyspnea and dysphagia may occur. There is a higher frequency of concurrent other autoimmune disorders, which may also occur among other family members.

LINEAR SCLERODERMA

This is the most frequent form of childhood LSc. Linear bands of sclerosis occur on limbs or face and may overlie the joints or scalp, respectively (Figures 8.4 and 8.5). The distribution is usually transverse over the trunk (Figure 8.6) and longitudinal on the limbs (Figure 8.7) and face (Figure 8.8). It has a chronic relapsing course with

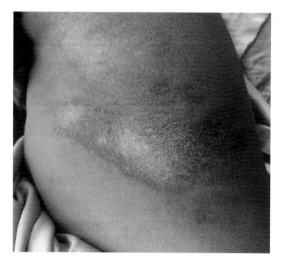

Figure 8.1 Lilac-colored plaque of morphea; central atrophy is observed at the lower part of the lesion.

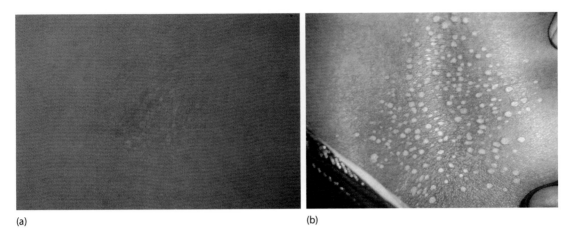

(a)   (b)

Figure 8.3 (**a, b**) Multiple subcentimetric hypo-pigmented papules of guttate morphea in a child (**a**) and in an adult (**b**).

various complications, like joint contracture, claw hands (Figure 8.9) or hammer toes, limb length discrepancies, and atrophy of the underlying deeper tissues.

Linear scleroderma involving the face and scalp is also termed as *en coup de sabre* (Figure 8.10). It is unilateral and may also affect the underlying bone (Figure 8.11) and other organs causing seizures, uveitis, and other ocular and dental abnormalities. Cicatricial alopecia of the eyelashes, eyebrows, or scalp may occur if the lesion overlies these areas. Parry-Romberg syndrome is the progressive hemifacial atrophy (Figure 8.12) involving mainly the lower face with minimal or no skin surface

changes. The absence of inflammation and sclerosis prior to the severe atrophy in Parry-Romberg syndrome prompt some researchers to consider it as a separate entity, and it is a close differential diagnosis of *en coup de sabre*,

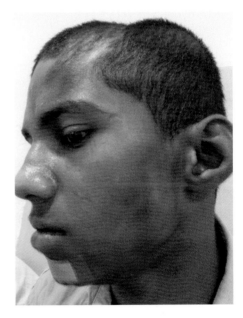

Figure 8.5 Linear scleroderma involving left side of face, extending to scalp, resulting in atrophy and loss of hair.

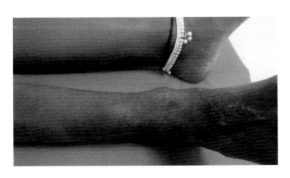

Figure 8.4 Linear scleroderma with atrophy and sclerosis on lower limb overlying the ankle joint.

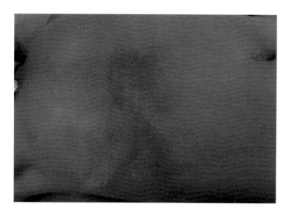

Figure 8.6 Linear scleroderma involving right half of body (same child as in Figure 8.4) with transverse distribution of the lesion on trunk.

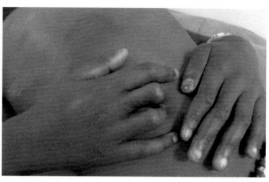

Figure 8.9 Claw hand on right side in a child with linear scleroderma.

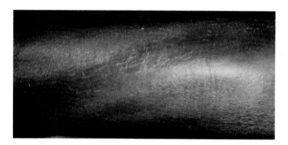

Figure 8.7 Hyper-pigmented, atrophic band of linear morphea on limb.

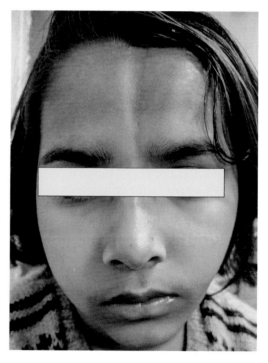

Figure 8.10 *En coup de Sabre.*

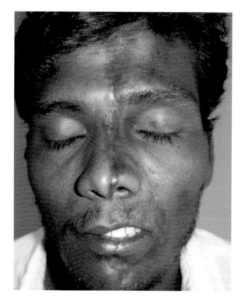

Figure 8.8 Linear morphea on the face of an adult patient; there is atrophy of the upper lip and loss of moustache on the involved area.

PANSCLEROTIC MORPHEA

In this least common type but most severe variant of childhood LSc, fibrosis is confined to the deep dermis. Owing to the inconsistency of the reported literature on the depth of involvement, recently, it has been defined as the "presence of near total body surface area involvement with

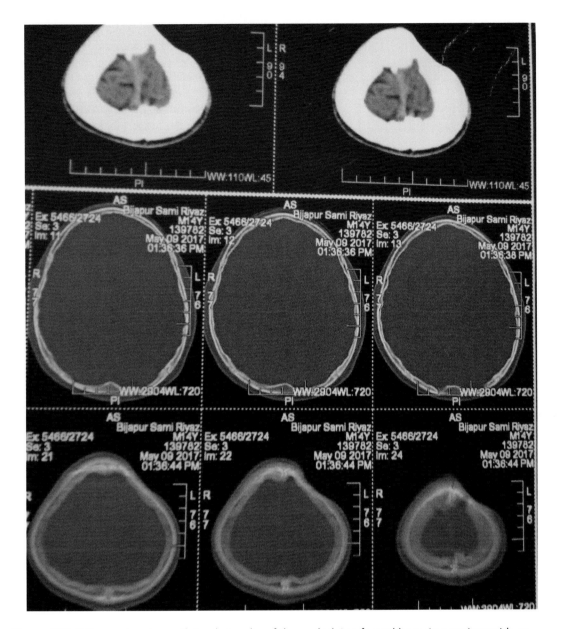

Figure 8.11 CT scan showing unilateral atrophy of the underlying frontal bone in a patient with *en coup de Sabre*.

sparing of the fingers and toes." It is frequently complicated by severe joint contractures, chronic ulcerations, and development of squamous cell carcinoma.

MIXED VARIANT

It is a condition in which a combination of two or more of the other subtypes of morphea coexists in the same patient. It accounts for around 20% of the pediatric LSc.

EXTRACUTANEOUS MANIFESTATIONS

Around a quarter of children affected with LSc may develop one or more extra-cutaneous manifestation during the course of their disease. A few may progress to SSc. Compared to adults, who may

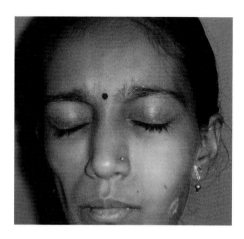

Figure 8.12 Parry-Romberg syndrome with right hemifacial atrophy.

show associated autoimmune disorders in around 30%, only 5% of the children with LSc show such associations.[2] These are common in generalized and mixed variants.

Extracutaneous manifestations in patients with LSc include arthritis, neurological, ocular, gastrointestinal, and pulmonary changes.[3] An extensive evaluation for these associations is indicated in the presence of clinical suspicion and positive antibody profile.

Arthritis: Joint involvement is the most frequent association with LSc present in a quarter of the patients. It is seen especially in linear morphea and often associated with a positive rheumatoid factor (RF). These children tend to have a rapid course of the disease with a high propensity for contractures.

Neurologic features: Seizures and headaches are the most frequent neurologic associations. However, neuro-psychiatric disabilities have also been described. A headache may be the presenting sign of *en coup de sabre*. Apart from these clinical findings, radiological changes like calcifications, white matter changes, vascular malformations, and vasculitis-like changes have also been demonstrated.[4]

Eye changes: Ocular changes have been documented in around 3% of childhood LSc, the majority being in *en coup de sabre* variant affecting the face. These include adnexal changes, anterior segment inflammation,

central nervous system (CNS) abnormalities, refractive errors, and rarely strabismus.[5]

Gastrointestinal changes: Esophageal motor function abnormalities with gastro-esophageal reflux and associated esophagitis are the common gastrointestinal findings seen in childhood LSc, similar to the adults.

Pulmonary changes: Restrictive type of respiratory difficulty with a mild decrease in respiratory volume and impaired diffusing capacity of the lungs have been reported with childhood LSc.

JUVENILE SYSTEMIC SCLEROSIS

In children, most patients have the diffuse cutaneous-type SSc (dSSc), and the localized cutaneous SSc (lcSSc) is uncommon. Only one case of childhood scleroderma-*sine*-scleroderma has been reported,[6] and there are no reports of environmentally induced scleroderma in childhood. In patients less than 16 years of age, JSSc is diagnosed when the major criterion of proximal sclerosis/induration of the skin and 2 out of 20 minor criteria have been satisfied.[7]

Epidemiology

Children constitute only less than 5% of all systemic sclerosis cases, in general. Moreover, 5%–10% of adult cases of systemic sclerosis develop the disease before the age of 18 years.

Clinical features

The onset of JSSc is usually insidious, and the interval between onset and diagnosis in childhood is often long. Following onset, the course may be prolonged with alternate periods of active and inactive disease. A majority present with skin tightening and or Raynaud's phenomenon (RP). Other features include joint and muscle pain, subcutaneous calcification, dyspnea, and dysphagia.

Cutaneous features are as follows:

GENERAL FEATURES

Edema of the hands and feet is the initial manifestation followed by a gradually progressive cutaneous sclerosis. Soon hands become shiny with tapering fingertips. Taut facial skin results in masking of minute expressions from muscle movements giving rise to characteristic emotionless facies. The forehead is shiny without wrinkling on looking up, pinched nose, decreased oral aperture, and loss of volume of the lips and gingiva resulting in prominence of teeth. There are mat-like telangiectasia on bilateral cheeks. Patients often complain of an increase in pigmentation before the onset of scleroderma. In later phases, patchy "salt and pepper" pigmentation is appreciable. Calcinosis cutis, especially at the distal areas that often leave refractory ulcers, may also develop in long-standing cases.

Raynaud's phenomenon (RP): Even though RP is uncommon in the pediatric population, it is the presenting feature of JSSc in up to 70% cases. It has a characteristic triad of pallor due to vasoconstriction, cyanosis due to reduced oxygen saturation, followed by redness due to reactive hyperemia; often precipitated by cold or emotional stimuli. Sometimes the sites may be ears, tip of nose, tongue, lips, and cheeks and the symptoms may be numbness, tingling sensation, pain, and localized hyperhidrosis.

Nailfold capillary changes: Typical microvascular changes of JSSc can be easily assessed by the characteristic nailfold capillary changes associated with it. Apart from differentiating primary RP from secondary RP by the absence of nailfold capillary changes, it also mirrors the ongoing activity and extent of systemic involvement in JSSc. The scleroderma pattern of capillary changes includes an "early" pattern (i.e., few enlarged/giant capillaries, few capillary hemorrhages, no evident loss of capillaries), an "active" pattern (i.e., frequent giant capillaries, frequent capillary hemorrhages, mild disorganization of the capillary network), and a "late" pattern (i.e., irregular enlargement of the capillaries, few or absent giant capillaries, hemorrhages, and extensive avascular areas). According to a recent study, a typical scleroderma pattern may not be observed in up to 13% of the children with JSSc.[8] They were also less likely to suffer from dSSc subtype, ANA and Scl-70 positivity, digital ulcers, and joint contractures.[8] Of those who showed a scleroderma pattern on capillaroscopy, an "early" or "active" pattern

signified an initial disease and minimal involvement of internal organs, and the "late" pattern was associated with later stages of the disease with significant internal organ involvement.[8] The correlation of distribution of these pattern subsets and clinical disease activity or extent of organ involvement was similar to adult-onset SSc.[8] However, JSSc patients were found to display a scleroderma pattern more frequently compared to adult-onset SSc (93.3% versus 87.8%).[9]

Organ involvement is less common in JSSc as compared to adult-onset SSc. Arthritis and myositis may occur in one-third of the children with JSSc, and the arthralgia may be a presenting symptom in 15% of the patients. Gastrointestinal involvement is reported in up to three-quarters of the patients of JSSc during their disease course. In addition to the common complaints of gastro-esophageal reflux disease and dysphagia due to lower esophageal sphincter involvement, large bowel involvement may present with constipation, diarrhea, bloating, and malabsorption.

Pulmonary involvement in the form of interstitial lung disease is rarely reported in children, unlike in adults. Since the lung involvement is usually asymptomatic and may present as dry cough or frank dyspnoea when the fibrosis develops, pulmonary function testing helps in early detection of the lung involvement. Severe pulmonary involvement also results in cardiac complications. JSSc *per se* may result in cardiac fibrosis, myocarditis, resultant arrhythmias, and ventricular dysfunctions. Around 10% of the JSSc children may show abnormal renal parameters. However, less than 5% develop renal failure and only less than 1% develop scleroderma renal crisis.

Even though rare, cardiac involvement portends a bad prognosis with fatal congestive cardiac failure, arrhythmias, and sudden cardiac death. The cardiac manifestation that includes myocardial fibrosis, or hypertrophy, and conduction abnormalities often begins early in the disease course and remain clinically asymptomatic. Only subclinical cardiovascular changes were noted in adult patients with juvenile-onset scleroderma.[10] Significant echocardiographic changes were noted in patients with associated musculoskeletal and organ involvement as well as immunological positivity for anti-Scl-70.[11]

Table 8.1 Differentiating features between LSc and JSSc (lcSSc and dSSc)

Feature	LSc	lcJSSc	dcJSSc
Immunological markers	Usually negative	ANA+ in 80%–97% Anticentromere ab+ in <10%	Anti-topoisomerase I (Scl-70) ab+ 20%–30%
Skin involvement	Localized areas	Face and acral areas	Extends to proximal limbs and trunks
Progression	Slow, except in generalized morphea	Slower onset and progression	Rapid onset and progression
Raynaud's phenomenon	Absent	Long history of RP before skin involvement	Short history or concomitant RP along with skin involvement
Calcinosis	Absent	Frequent	May occur
Lung involvement	Absent	Primary pulmonary arterial hypertension (PAH), lung fibrosis infrequent	Lung fibrosis frequent, secondary PAH
Other organ involvement	Absent	Gastroesophageal reflux universal	Scleroderma renal crisis

Juvenile systemic sclerosis with limited cutaneous involvement

Limited cutaneous systemic sclerosis is less common in children than in adults. The sclerosis of the fingers not extending beyond the wrists is the classical finding in this variant. Calcinosis, RP, Esophageal dysmotility, Sclerodactyly, and Telangiectasia (CREST syndrome) typifies the manifestations of lcSSc. RP predates the skin involvement by years. The disease is usually slowly progressive with most of the patients having a benign course of the disease. Differences in the clinical presentations of LSc and JSSc (lcSSc and dSSc) have been given in Table 8.1.

DIAGNOSIS

Diagnosis of childhood scleroderma is based mainly on clinical features and a histopathology may be indicated when there is an ambiguity in clinical diagnosis. However, various clinical and laboratory tools have been introduced for the monitoring of the clinical activity discussed in other sections.

Localized Scleroderma Severity Index (LoSSI)[12] and the Localized Scleroderma Damage Index (LoSDI)[13] are the clinical scoring systems that score the 18 body parts based on skin thickness,

inflammation, lesion extension, and damage on a scale of 0 to 3. These highly subjective tests are not validated in large cohort of patients.

Around 40% patients are positive for anti-nuclear antibody (ANA) tests, while only 4% are positive for antibodies to double-stranded DNA (ds-DNA).[1] Antibodies to single-stranded DNA (ss-DNA) have been found to be positive in 20%–55% of LSc patients and well correlated with the extent of the disease. There are no specific serological markers available to evaluate the disease activity. Non-invasive tools like thermography, durometer, ultrasonography, laser Doppler flowmetry, and magnetic resonance imaging (MRI) have been increasingly used to assess the extent and, sometimes, the activity of the disease.

PROGNOSIS

Although the long-term studies on the prognosis of LSc and JSSc are meagre, the available evidence suggests that the disease runs a chronic and recurrent course that often results in sequelae.[14] Both methotrexate and systemic steroids tend to stop the progression of the disease in short-term; however, the disease recurs in up to 50% of the patients within two years of stopping the treatment.[15,16] Persistent activity was noted in 28%–89% of the patients in some other studies.[17,18] In a retrospective study of 52 patients with linear morphea, one-third had active disease after 10 years, all but one had aesthetic sequelae and up to 38% had functional impairment.[17] Individuals with LSc during childhood may have an impaired quality of life and are more likely to develop autoimmune diseases during adulthood.[18]

In general, the JSSc appears to have a better prognosis compared to the adult counterpart with a five-year survival of 95%. Cardiomyopathy is the leading cause of death in children. In adult-onset dcSSc, the presence of immune markers, like anti-topoisomerase I and anti-RNA polymerase III antibodies, and male gender are considered to be associated with a poorer prognosis. No such risk factors have been identified in JSSc.[19] However, the evidence of fibrosis on chest X-rays, raised creatinine levels, and pericarditis have been associated with a poor outcome in JSSc.

TREATMENT

There is no consensus on the treatment of pediatric scleroderma owing to the lack of well-conducted clinical trials in this disorder. Evidence of treatment for LSc is mainly based on case series and low-quality comparative trials. There is no recommended treatment guideline for JSSc either, and the management is based on the EULAR recommendation for adult SSc.

Treatment of localized scleroderma (LSc)

The treatment of LSc should be initiated at an earlier stage before complications occur due to restricted mobility and deformities. However, if only disease damage parameters exist, and clinical activity is absent, the simple monitoring of the lesion is recommended. It may be difficult to assess the disease activity, and the following features should be taken into consideration while assessing disease progression or stability;

- The appearance of new lesions in the last three months (documented by physician)
- Expansion of a pre-existing lesion in the last three months (documented by physician)
- Moderate or severe erythema or skin lesions with erythematous borders

- Violaceous hue on the surface of the lesion or at the border
- Increased induration at the border of the lesion.
- Worsening of hair loss on the scalp, eyebrows, or eyelashes (documented by physician)
- Documentation of disease activity or progression to deeper tissues (by photography, MRI or ultrasonography
- Increased creatine kinase in the absence of other changes
- Histopathological evidence of disease activity in skin

Except in generalized and linear morphea, topical therapy in the form of topical steroids, topical calcineurin inhibitors, topical vitamin-D analogs, and emollients are the mainstay of treatment.

Systemic therapy is indicated when there is a significant risk of morbidity, such as in deep pansclerotic morphea, progressive linear morphea overlying a joint, and generalized morphea. In these cases, evidence for methotrexate therapy is robust. The usual regimen is 1 mg/kg/week (up to a maximum of 25 mg/week) of methotrexate along with folic acid supplementation. The addition of systemic corticosteroids (methylprednisolone infusion; 30 mg/kg 3 consecutive days/month) or 0.5–1 mg/kg/day of oral prednisolone as an induction therapy during the initial three months improves the efficacy of the therapeutic regimen.[15,17] Phototherapy (low or medium dose UVA1, narrow-band UVB) or photo-chemotherapy (PUVA) have also been found to be efficacious in LSc.[14] Patients who do not tolerate or respond to these regimens can be started with mycophenolate mofetil at a dose of 500 to 1000 mg/m^2/day.[20]

TREATMENT OF JUVENILE SYSTEMIC SCLEROSIS (JSSc)

A number of immunosuppressive or immunomodulatory agents are used with varying success in SSc. Moreover, the treatment should also address the organ involvement associated with the disease. A summary of these treatment approaches has been detailed in Table 8.2.[21–29] Being a slowly progressive disease with the possibility of natural resolution of skin tethering, ascertaining the contribution of individual drugs used in various therapeutic trials of SSc is challenging. While systemic steroids, methotrexate, cyclophosphamide,

Table 8.2 Therapeutic options for JSSc

Indication	Drugs and dosage	Remarks
Immunomodulation	Mycophenolate mofetil (MMF), 1–3 g/day	Promising results for skin involvement and pulmonary fibrosis.
	Systemic steroids; Prednisolone, 10 mg/day	Long-term, high dose steroids may precipitate a renal crisis and hence not recommended.
		Indicated in the early edematous phase of skin involvement, myositis, arthritis, symptomatic serositis.
	Cyclophosphamide, 50–150 mg/day	Unknown efficacy as a single agent. Efficacious for fibrosing alveolitis when used in combination with systemic steroids.
	Methotrexate, 0.3–0.6 mg/kg/week	For skin involvement.
	Rituximab	Improvement of skin fibrosis and prevention of worsening lung fibrosis.
	Imatinib mesylate, 400 mg/day	Improvement in skin and lung fibrosis.
	Intravenous immunoglobulin, (IVIG), 2 g/kg	Improvement in skin fibrosis.
	Tocilizumab, 8–12 mg/kg, subcutaneous given at 0, 2, and 4 weeks and then at 4-weekly intervals	Improvement in skin fibrosis.
	Autologous hematopoietic stem cell transplantation (HSCT)	Efficacy in preventing disease progression.
Pruritus	Antihistamines Emollients	Low-dose oral glucocorticoids (less than 10 mg daily dose of prednisolone) may be needed for severe pruritus.
Telangiectasia	Camouflaged with make-up, Laser or other light therapy	
Calcinosis cutis	Diltiazem, 2–4 mg/kg/day Colchicine, 1 mg/day Minocycline, 50–100 mg/day Topical sodium thiosulfate or sodium metabisulfite Surgery	Colchicine and minocycline preferred for inflamed, ulcerated lesions. Other therapies include oral aluminium hydroxide, warfarin, bisphosphonates, and intralesional steroids.
Raynaud's phenomenon	Calcium channel blockers (CCBs) Intravenous prostanoids	Nifedipine, 0.2 mg/kg 8 hourly.
Digital ulcers	CCBs and prostanoids Bosentan	Potential liver injury and teratogenicity with Bosentan
Lung involvement	Steroids and cyclophosphamide	Low-dose prednisolone (0.2–0.4 mg/kg per day) and cyclophosphamide, either as a daily oral regimen (1–2 mg/kg per day) or as a monthly single intravenous pulse (500–750 mg/m² per month)

(Continued)

Table 8.2 (*Continued*) Therapeutic options for JSSc

Indication	Drugs and dosage	Remarks
Renal Disease	Angiotensin-converting enzyme (ACE) inhibitors	Prevention of vascular damage, effective long-term control of blood pressure, and stabilization of renal function.
Musculoskeletal involvement	Steroids, Prednisolone, 0.3–0.5 mg/kg/day	Potential increased risk of scleroderma renal crisis.
Gastrointestinal disease	Proton-pump inhibitors (PPIs) Antibiotics Nutritional supplements	PPIs for reflux disease and antibiotics for bacterial overgrowth under the supervision of a gastroenterologist.

and mycophenolate mofetil have been found to be useful in SSc based on larger studies, efficacy and safety of emerging treatments like rituximab and tocilizumab are yet to be substantiated.

REFERENCES

1. Zulian F, Athreya BH, Laxer R. et al. Juvenile localized scleroderma: Clinical and epidemiological features in 750 children. An international study. *Rheumatology (Oxford)*. 2006;45:614–620.
2. Leitenberger JJ, Cayce RL, Haley RW, Adams-Huet B, Bergstresser PR, Jacobe HT. Distinct autoimmune syndromes in morphea: A review of 245 adult and pediatric cases. *Arch Dermatol*. 2009;145:545–550.
3. Zulian F, Vallongo C, Woo P. et al. Localized scleroderma in childhood is not just a skin disease. *Arthritis Rheum* 2005;52:2873–2881.
4. Doolittle DA, Lehman VT, Schwartz KM, Wong-Kisiel LC, Lehman JS, Tollefson MM. CNS imaging findings associated with Parry-Romberg syndrome and en coup de sabre: Correlation to dermatologic and neurologic abnormalities. *Neuroradiology* 2015;57:21–34.
5. Zannin ME, Martini G, Athreya BH. et al. Ocular involvement in children with localised scleroderma: A multi-centre study. *Br J Ophthalmol*. 2007;91:1311–1314.
6. Navon P, Halevi A, Brand A, Branski D, Rubinow A. Progressive systemic sclerosis sine scleroderma in a child presenting as nocturnal seizures and Raynaud's phenomenon. *Acta Paediatr* 1993;82:122–123.
7. Zulian F, Woo P, Athreya BH. et al. The Pediatric Rheumatology European Society/American College of Rheumatology/European League against Rheumatism provisional classification criteria for juvenile systemic sclerosis. *Arthritis Rheum* 2007;57:203–212.
8. Ingegnoli F, Ardoino I, Boracchi P, Cutolo M. Nailfold capillaroscopy in systemic sclerosis: Data from the EULAR scleroderma trials and research (EUSTAR) database. *Microvasc Res* 2013;89:122–128.
9. Ingegnoli F, Boracchi P, Gualtierotti R, Smith V, Cutolo M, Foeldvari I. A comparison between nailfold capillaroscopy patterns in adulthood in juvenile and adult-onset systemic sclerosis: A EUSTAR exploratory study. *Microvasc Res* 2015;102:19–24.
10. Borowiec A, Dabrowski R, Wozniak J. et al. Cardiovascular assessment of asymptomatic patients with juvenile-onset localized and systemic scleroderma: 10 years prospective observation. *Scand J Rheumatol* 2012;41:33–38.
11. Dedeoglu R, Adrovic A, Oztunc F, Sahin S, Barut K, Kasapcopur O. New insights into cardiac involvement in juvenile scleroderma: A three-dimensional echo-cardiographic assessment unveils subclinical ventricle dysfunction. *Pediatr Cardiol* 2017;38:1686–1695.
12. Arkachaisri T, Vilaiyuk S, Li S. et al. The localized scleroderma skin severity index and physician global assessment of disease activity: A work in progress toward development of localized scleroderma outcome measures. *J Rheumatol* 2009;36:2819–2829.

13. Arkachaisri T, Vilaiyuk S, Torok KS, Medsger TA, Jr. Development and initial validation of the localized scleroderma skin damage index and physician global assessment of disease damage: A proof-of-concept study. *Rheumatology (Oxford)* 2010;49:373–381.

14. Aranegui B, Jimenez-Reyes J. Morphea in childhood: An update. *Actas Dermosifiliogr* 2018;109:312–322.

15. Zulian F, Martini G, Vallongo C. et al. Methotrexate treatment in juvenile localized scleroderma: A randomized, double-blind, placebo-controlled trial. *Arthritis Rheum* 2011;63:1998–2006.

16. Mirsky L, Chakkittakandiyil A, Laxer RM, O'Brien C, Pope E. Relapse after systemic treatment in paediatric morphoea. *Br J Dermatol* 2012;166:443–445.

17. Piram M, McCuaig CC, Saint-Cyr C. et al. Short- and long-term outcome of linear morphoea in children. *Br J Dermatol* 2013;169:1265–1271.

18. Saxton-Daniels S, Jacobe HT. An evaluation of long-term outcomes in adults with pediatric-onset morphea. *Arch Dermatol* 2010;146:1044–1045.

19. Martini G, Vittadello F, Kasapcopur O. et al. Factors affecting survival in juvenile systemic sclerosis. *Rheumatology (Oxford)* 2009;48:119–122.

20. Martini G, Ramanan AV, Falcini F, Girschick H, Goldsmith DP, Zulian F. Successful treatment of severe or methotrexate-resistant juvenile localized scleroderma with mycophenolate mofetil. *Rheumatology (Oxford)* 2009;48:1410–1413.

21. Herrick AL, Pan X, Peytrignet S. et al. Treatment outcome in early diffuse cutaneous systemic sclerosis: The European Scleroderma Observational Study (ESOS). *Ann Rheum Dis* 2017;76:1207–1218.

22. Tashkin DP, Roth MD, Clements PJ. et al. Mycophenolate mofetil versus oral cyclophosphamide in scleroderma-related interstitial lung disease (SLS II): A randomised controlled, double-blind, parallel group trial. *Lancet Respir Med* 2016;4:708–719.

23. Valentini G, Paone C, La Montagna G. et al. Low-dose intravenous cyclophosphamide in systemic sclerosis: An open prospective efficacy study in patients with early diffuse disease. *Scand J Rheumatol* 2006;35:35–38.

24. Kowal-Bielecka O, Landewe R, Avouac J. et al. EULAR recommendations for the treatment of systemic sclerosis: A report from the EULAR Scleroderma Trials and Research group (EUSTAR). *Ann Rheum Dis* 2009;68:620–628.

25. Jordan S, Distler JH, Maurer B. et al. Effects and safety of rituximab in systemic sclerosis: An analysis from the European Scleroderma Trial and Research (EUSTAR) group. *Ann Rheum Dis* 2015;74:1188–1194.

26. Spiera RF, Gordon JK, Mersten JN. et al. Imatinib mesylate (Gleevec) in the treatment of diffuse cutaneous systemic sclerosis: Results of a 1-year, phase IIa, single-arm, open-label clinical trial. *Ann Rheum Dis* 2011;70:1003–1009.

27. Sullivan KM, Goldmuntz EA, Keyes-Elstein L. et al. Myeloablative autologous stem-cell transplantation for severe scleroderma. *N Engl J Med* 2018;378:35–47.

28. Poelman CL, Hummers LK, Wigley FM, Anderson C, Boin F, Shah AA. Intravenous immunoglobulin may be an effective therapy for refractory, active diffuse cutaneous systemic sclerosis. *J Rheumatol* 2015;42:236–242.

29. Lythgoe H, Baildam E, Beresford MW, Cleary G, McCann LJ, Pain CE. Tocilizumab as a potential therapeutic option for children with severe, refractory juvenile localized scleroderma. *Rheumatology (Oxford)* 2018;57:398–401.

Index

Note: Page numbers in italic and bold refer to figures and tables respectively.